Nicolas Scheffer
Jean-Philippe Lang

Substance use and creativity

Application in the treatment of addictions

ScienciaScripts

Imprint

Any brand names and product names mentioned in this book are subject to trademark, brand or patent protection and are trademarks or registered trademarks of their respective holders. The use of brand names, product names, common names, trade names, product descriptions etc. even without a particular marking in this work is in no way to be construed to mean that such names may be regarded as unrestricted in respect of trademark and brand protection legislation and could thus be used by anyone.

Cover image: www.ingimage.com

This book is a translation from the original published under ISBN 978-620-2-28820-0.

Publisher:
Sciencia Scripts
is a trademark of
Dodo Books Indian Ocean Ltd. and OmniScriptum S.R.L publishing group

120 High Road, East Finchley, London, N2 9ED, United Kingdom
Str. Armeneasca 28/1, office 1, Chisinau MD-2012, Republic of Moldova, Europe
Printed at: see last page
ISBN: 978-620-5-93980-2

Table of contents

1. Introduction

If the idea that psychoactive substances and artistic creation are linked has crossed our minds as readers or spectators of works of art, this work has as a starting point a clinical reflection and as a thread a point of view and hopefully a medical rigor. It originates from a conversation with a doctor who noticed that he had several active artists, living from their work, among the patients he treated for addiction problems. We wondered together about the existence of a link, about the impact of their treatment on their profession, about the impact of their profession on their treatment, and the idea of exploring these issues further seemed interesting. The different people we consulted afterwards to gather their ideas were enthusiastic and after a few months, our subject crystallized. On the one hand we have art, creativity, creation, and on the other hand, psychoactive substances and addictions to these substances. Are these two poles linked? Can they be? In what way? What are the consequences in medicine? We quickly realized the difficulty of the undertaking and in particular the difficulty of framing the research.

We are thus in the presence of two poles, two domains, which can be seen as two protagonists, and our first objective is to get to know them better before making them intersect. This is the aim of our first three parts, which from this point of view are coherent: to explore, collect and organize information. We wanted to multiply the angles of approach, which explains why we devoted an entire part to pleasure. This part allowed us a more philosophical approach and thus a better understanding of our subject. In the same way, we have systematically adopted a psychodynamic and neurobiological point of view in addition to a more general one. The complexity and the sometimes abstruse character of these disciplines did not make our task easy. The data provided will therefore appear, perhaps, a little blurred or trivial to specialists, but we did not want to leave these areas aside. Finally, we have to accept that all this information will not be oriented towards a goal, towards a demonstration; this is undoubtedly linked to the exploratory and creative nature of our work.

Now that we know more about the protagonists, we will try to find out what kind of relationship they may have. The first possibility is that of mutual influence. The idea is that if one is there, the other is more likely to be there. We have two hypotheses. First, the psychoactive substances encourage the artist to experiment or continue using. This influence can be on the core of the creative process (directly or indirectly), but also on the person and their environment (consumer expectations and inspiration). Secondly, a person, because he is an artist, will be encouraged in his consumption: artistic creation will lead to consumption. This hypothesis is underpinned by psychological (creation generates anxiety) and socio-cultural (living conditions and the influence of myth) explanations.

Once we have considered these mutual influences, we will turn to another type of relationship. The idea is that both protagonists are there for the same reasons and have the same missions, "common roots and wings". Substance use and artistic creation have causes and consequences in common. We will see first of all that psychological characteristics, psychopathological or events, can constitute common roots. We will then see that if the processes are quite different, their functions are essential, diverse and partly common: to modify our emotions, to alleviate our sufferings, to envisage death and the emptiness of the existence, and to seek pleasure and joy.

After having, we hope, better understood the relationship between psychoactive substances and artistic creation, we will try to draw an idea for practice and in particular for addiction problems. The common roots and functions mentioned above, suggest on the one hand that artistic creation can *contribute to fulfilling* the functions of addictive practices, and on the other hand that artistic practices can *help to acquire skills* to fulfill these functions, with or without art.

In practice, it is in the artistic mediation therapies that these ideas can be found. We have therefore looked in the scientific literature for applications of this type of therapy to addiction problems. Different axes of work emerge: expression, communication, the place of emotions, defenses, the feeling of control and self-esteem. We will then discuss the variety of theoretical frameworks and practical modalities before presenting some results.

This is the broad outline of the work we propose. We hope that it will help to clarify the links between psychoactive substances and creativity. In the field of addiction treatment, it will bring arguments in favor of the use of artistic practices, in a therapeutic framework.

2. Creativity

2.1. . General

Why choose the term creativity? It is a fashionable term, of recent appearance in the French language (it still appears in quotation marks in the 1950s), a somewhat vague term, which covers a vast and difficult to define domain... a term that is not very engaging. So why this choice? The term creativity has the advantage of focusing on the individual, on the artist and on the genesis of the work. Most of the articles we have studied use this word and it therefore seemed legitimate to us to retain it.

We will also use the term creation. Creativity seems to correspond more to a potential, an attitude, a way of apprehending things and even life in general. In "the body of the work"[1] D. Anzieu assimilates creativity to a propulsion, to a horizontal force and speaks of creation as a take-off.

2.1.1. . Definition

The dictionary of the French Academy tells us: "derived from creative, ability to create, to invent". If we look in the Larousse, we can add the capacity of "imagination", that is to say "the capacity to elaborate new images and conceptions, to find original solutions to problems". We touch on the first characteristic of creativity: the ability to produce something new, different, original. A second characteristic seems to be agreed upon. A random process can generate novelty but something is missing: an adapted, useful aspect. Thus creativity is usually defined as requiring both originality and utility.[2]

2.1.2. . Different areas

Is creativity different depending on the domain in which it is exercised?[3] Studies that assess products lean toward domain specificity while those assessing individuals lean toward generality across domains. Models attempt to unify the two views[4]; of general and domain-specific skills certainly coexist.

2.1.3. . Different levels

It is clear that there is a gradation in creativity. To clarify things and to frame the research, categories have been created. "Big-C": major, eminent creativity and "little-c", everyday creativity.[3] " Mini-c" corresponds to creativity felt only by its author, very subjective, and delimits the lower field of the "little- c" category. "Pro-C" is a category between "little" and "big" and corresponds, for example, to a professional artist who has not reached the status of a recognized artist.[5]

2.2. . The Process

2.2.1. . Many mental processes and several models

Creation is mysterious. It is attributed to a "genius", to an inner force that guides and inspires the artist. J. P Guilford has made considerable progress in the study of creativity. As president of the American Psychological Association in 1949, he called for the study of creativity, arguing that a very small percentage of the literature was devoted to this subject, and that its understanding required scientific methods and could contribute much to society as a whole. His work on the structure of the intellect led to the identification of the concept of divergent thinking, which is essential for the evaluation of creativity.

In practice, we examine the ability to answer open-ended questions, without a specific answer. For example, if we ask the question: "What can you do with a brick?", or "What would happen if you didn't need sleep?", we can give a large number of answers, without any of them being THE right answer (alternative use test). The number of answers corresponds to fluency and the number of different categories mentioned corresponds to flexibility. Originality is measured in relation to the answers given to this question in the general population, and elaboration is the ability to develop the answers given. On this basis, one of the most popular creativity "tests" has been developed: the Torrance Test of Creative Thinking, which measures each of these four components in two categories: verbal and figurative.

Mednick[6] insisted that the reason we move from one idea to another is because they are associated in our minds in some way, and that creative people are good at associating distant ideas.

Besides association, other useful mental processes have been identified. Without being exhaustive, we can mention the creation of mental images, conceptual combination, analogies, metaphors, restructuring, definition of a problem...

Wallas developed a model[7] that is still widely used, according to which four phases follow one another: preparation, incubation, illumination and verification. Preparation corresponds to the identification and definition of the problem and the objective, and the gathering of knowledge. Incubation is the unconscious cognitive process. Intimation (often considered a sub-stage) corresponds to the feeling that the solution is on its way. Illumination is the stage where the solution, the idea, "arrives" in our mind. Verification is the confrontation of the solution with reality. Back and forth can take place between these different phases.

Differences can be observed between cultures. Of course the language used is of great importance for the associations between ideas, but the culture "in general" also has an influence.[8]

2.2.2. . Neurobiology: a lack of theoretical coherence

Despite the few elements of consensus definition that we have presented, we do not have a single global model of creativity. Creativity seems to involve a large number of factors and most articles studying the neurobiology of creativity actually study the neurobiology of these different factors. A few elements seem to stand out: the centrality of the frontal cortex, the hypotheses on disinhibition, on excitation and on catecholamines.

In a review of the structures involved in creative cognition, we find both increases and decreases in substance (in volume and integrity) in different brain areas, changes that correlate with increased performance on creativity tests. These areas are scattered and may correspond to the "default mode network". A neural process of disinhibition within this network would be responsible for the creation of novelty and other exciting processes based on the "cognitive control network" would be responsible for the selective retention of certain elements produced (Blind Variation and Selective Retention model).[9]

In another review[10] , this time using electroencephalographic explorations, creative cognition processes are reflected by an increase in alpha power, i.e., an increase in alpha synchronization or an absence of alpha desynchronization (particularly at the frontal and posterior right parietal level). This would correspond to an inwardly oriented attention, to a processing of information not driven by stimuli or even to an inhibition of external stimuli.

Concerning the study of brain lesions, damage to the frontal lobes, and in particular the medial part of the prefrontal cortex, is traditionally associated with decreases in creativity and difficulties in divergent thinking[11] . Some studies have noted the importance of brain asymmetry. Lesions of the right hemisphere seemed to have a greater negative impact on creativity. Lesions of the left parietal cortex and the left inferior frontal gyrus seemed to be associated with greater originality. There may be competition between right and left fronto-parietal structures, which explains why these left lesions would relax the right structures and thus increase creativity.

Finally, the administration of L-Dopa (100mg L-Dopa and 25mg Benserazide) would increase the signal-to-noise ratio (evidenced by a decrease in the effects of indirect priming during a lexical decision test), which is related to a decrease in creativity (decrease in the association between words, distant ideas).[12]

2.2.3. . Psychoanalysis: sublimation, crisis and attitude towards the world

We will first explain the concept of sublimation. According to

According to Laplanche and Pontalis, it is a "process postulated by Freud to account for human activities apparently unrelated to sexuality, but which find their source in the strength of the sexual drive. Freud described as sublimation activities mainly artistic activity and intellectual investigation. The drive is said to be sublimated insofar as it is diverted to a new, non-sexual goal and aims at socially valued objects."[13]

In the inaugural chapter of a book devoted to artistic creation: "The body of the work"[1] , D. Anzieu explains that "to create requires, as a first condition, a symbolic filiation with a recognized creator. Without this filiation and without its subsequent denial, no paternity of a work is possible. Icarus always owes his wings to some maze. For him it is Freud, as for Freud it is Goethe. He also explains that the creation is a phase of crisis for the psychic apparatus, just like the mourning and the dream, which he calls a mini-crisis.

He then outlines the five phases of the creative process. Firstly, a state of seizure (allowing an inner crisis/dissociation/regression to occur), secondly, an awareness of unconscious material (unconscious psychic representative), then thirdly, these uncovered unconscious representatives/products/processes form a code, a code that allows reality (inner and outer) to be decoded and a work generated. Fourthly, there is a phase of work of composition of the work with compromises, unconscious defense mechanisms and finally, fifthly, an effect on the public.

Finally, for Winnicott, creativity seems to have a very general character: thus in "play and reality"[14] he writes: "The reader will agree, I hope, to consider creativity in its broadest sense, without confining it to the limits of a successful or recognized creation, but rather considering it as the coloring of any attitude towards external reality", he specifies that "it is above all a creative mode of perception which gives the individual the feeling that life is worth living; what opposes such a mode of perception is a relationship of submissive complacency towards external reality: the world and all its elements are then recognized but only as that to which one must adjust and adapt."

This creativity has its origin in the relationship of the child with his mother in his earliest childhood: "For Winnicott the capacity to live creatively, but also the original localization of cultural experience, are jointly articulated in this experience of keeping his mother in mind. (...) It is because "the sufficiently good mother" is capable of adapting to the needs of the child, that she authorizes and organizes a field of experience that allows the child to experience what is in the register of the transitional area, of creativity, and of what will become culture"[15]

The theory of the "Borromean knot" of Lacan allows to consider the artistic practice as a means to link, to tie the Real, the Symbolic and the Imaginary.

2.3. . The people

What makes one person more inclined or gifted than another to create, imagine, something? We will talk about some of the many factors that come into play.

2.3.1. . The personality

When we refer to personality, we are talking about "the set of affective, emotional, dynamic, relatively stable and general characteristics of a person's way of being in order to react to a situation in which he or she finds himself or herself.[16] Most often we reason in terms of personality traits. Various meta-analyses and reviews of the literature exist[17,18] . On the cognitive level, it is openness to experience that stands out very clearly in terms of its association with creativity.

Extraversion could also be correlated but only in certain sub-categories, and biased by the fact that creativity is often studied in groups. On the social level, we find the rejection of the norm, of tradition, of conservatism, which seems consistent with the definition of creativity. On the motivational level, it is both ambition and impulse that seem to be the most important traits.

Runco presents in his review of the literature[19] other personality traits, characteristics and tendencies: autonomy, flexibility, preference for complexity, openness to experience, sensitivity, playfulness, tolerance for ambiguity, risk-taking and risk tolerance, intrinsic motivation, psychological androgyny, self-efficacy, curiosity. He insists on the fact that these elements (which are not all "traits" per se) vary from one domain to another, interacting. They have an optimum (idea of moderation). Some are socially valued, others less so or not.

2.3.2. . The role of the family

The family has an important role in the development of creativity, as shown by the concentration of geniuses in certain families. Genetic factors, others related to education or more broadly to the environment can be advanced. It should be noted that the development of creativity is bidirectional, parents can stimulate their children's creativity and conversely children can stimulate their parents' creativity.

Studies have looked at parental variables: not surprisingly, parental creativity is predictive of children's creativity. On a dynamic level, the relationships with parents and family members are determining factors. The style of education was also analyzed and it was noted, for example, that a certain amount of independence given to children at an early age stimulates their creativity.[19]

The economic and social factors influencing creativity are exercised within the family and are modulated by it: multiplication of experiences (some of which will be "crystallizing"), trips, cultural outings are all possibilities to develop children's creativity.

Finally, family structure is particularly important. Family size seems to enhance creativity, as does being the second child. The loss of family members also has a considerable impact. If the death of the father often causes the birth of the work, if the disappearance of the mother haunts the work like a permanent wound, the loss of an elder brother or sister before his or her own birth is also heavy with consequences. Thus the fact of being a "replacement child", as in the case of Camille Claudel, contributes to explain the exceptional creativity of certain artists.[20]

2.3.3. . Psychiatric disorders

The first study using a scientific method on the links between creation and psychiatric disorders was conducted by Nancy C. Andreasen[21] . She studied 30 writers who were members of the University of Iowa Writers Workshop. 80% of the writers had an affective disorder compared to 30% of the controls, 43% had bipolar disorder compared to 10% of the controls and 30% had alcoholism compared to 7% of the controls. These three items were the only ones that were statistically significant. In particular, intelligence measured by the Wechsler Adult Intelligence

Scale (WAIS) did not vary between the two groups. Both creativity (literary and otherwise) and psychiatric pathology appeared to be overrepresented in the writers' families, especially the siblings.

A Scandinavian study[22] more recently studied the national register of the Swedish population, comprising more than one million people. The results do not find any association between psychopathology and creative occupation, neither scientific nor artistic, except for bipolar disorders for artists. The association is even generally negative. For the authors' sub-population, on the other hand, a clear association was found for most psychiatric disorders.

2.3.4. . The mood

Without going into the context of bipolar disorder, the effects of mood on creativity have been widely studied.[23] A positive mood is thought to lead to greater creativity than a neutral mood. The results do not seem to converge for comparisons between negative and neutral moods, although correlation studies find an association between anxiety, fear and low flexibility. Still in the same meta-analysis, a third category of studies comparing positive and negative moods did not find any significant difference.

The effects of mood on creativity seem difficult to characterize and the inclusion of arousal is necessary. It is important to include the idea of arousal in this type of study, but a detailed analysis of the effect of the product of mood and arousal on creativity seems difficult to carry out because of the lack of studies including states of serenity, relaxation or, on the contrary, anger. Still in the same review, mood should be put in perspective with the "regulatory focus", promotion or prevention, to better understand the effects of mood on creativity. To summarize, a positive mood could slightly improve creative abilities, but crises and a negative mood can be an important driver to move from potential to creation.

2.3.5. . Intelligence

Already in Alfred Binet's early tests, some questions assessing intelligence tested divergent thinking. It was found[18,24] that creativity tests and intelligence tests were only weakly or not at all correlated. The threshold theory[25] is commonly accepted. Below a certain intelligence, as measured in the classical way, creativity is difficult; above that, there is a creative potential, which is not necessarily realized. Intelligence would thus be necessary but not sufficient.

2.3.6. . Somatic disorders

Illnesses can lead to losses in abilities that are detrimental to creativity. For example, influenza reduces creativity test scores, particularly preference for complexity, in three quarters of those tested in a 1990 study[26] .

However, the most widespread idea is that of a beneficial effect of diseases or accidents on the creative path of individuals. In particular during childhood, these events can be creative turning points. We can cite many examples: Frida Kalho, Toulouse-Lautrec, Matisse... In adulthood, illnesses generate stress, pain, handicaps, which force artists to make changes that can result in an evolution of themes, style or even a change of technique (Degas, Dürer).[27]

2.4. . The environment

A person may be intelligent, motivated, and have a personality that is conducive to creation, but he or she must be in a favorable environment to be able to create something. A certain number of elements can be identified[28] All people do not react in the same way, and for example competition and stress can stimulate some people and inhibit others.

Another way to see this role of the environment is to study the history of art, to study in particular the social and cultural conditions that have allowed or favored artistic movements or remarkable creations.

3. The pleasure

Pleasure is not, strictly speaking, part of the title of our subject and yet we wanted to devote a chapter to it. If pleasure is a familiar and necessary concept to every human being, it seemed to us sometimes imprecise, vague. By defining it and by presenting some elements of reflection, we hope to take a step back and to clarify more precisely the relations between creation and use of psychoactive substances by placing them in a deeper universal process.

3.1. 1. General

"Nature has placed humanity under the government of two sovereign masters, pain and pleasure. It is to them alone that it belongs to signify what we should do, as well as to determine what we will do. On the one hand, the model of good and evil, on the other the chain of causes and effects, are riveted to their throne. They direct us in everything we do, in everything we say, in everything we think: any effort we might make to free ourselves from our subjection, will only serve to underline and confirm it. In words, a man may pretend to abjure their empire: but in reality, he will remain their subject forever."

J.Bentham[29]

3.1.1.1. Definition

The National Center for Textual and Literary Resources offers a definition of pleasure: "A pleasant, lasting emotional state created by the satisfaction of a need or desire or the accomplishment of a rewarding activity. The Larousse: "State of contentment created in someone by the satisfaction of a tendency, a need, a desire." Le dictionnaire de l'académie française (9th edition): "Impression that is created by what pleases, pleasure that one finds in the accomplishment of something. Sensation, pleasant emotion; feeling of contentment or well-being. Enjoyment, satisfaction of desire."

In "The Universal Philosophical Encyclopedia"[30] we find: "Movement or pleasant feeling that the soul experiences on the occasion of a physical or moral impression. A sensual pleasure is a pleasure, amusements or diversions are pleasures, but we can as well take pleasure in acts or thoughts. All living beings seek pleasure and shun pain". In the great dictionary of philosophy[31] : " Pleasant feeling that accompanies a sensation or an action, in the satisfaction of a need or the representation of a desire. Its variability shows that it is due to the meeting between a physical experience and an experience of freedom."

From these few definitions, we see that it is a state/sensation/feeling/impression/emotion that refers to something pleasant, satisfaction, enjoyment, contentment, well-being. Pleasure seems to be linked to desires or needs. It seems to be a driving force for man, attracted by this positive pole as it tends to move away from its opposite: displeasure and its corollaries: suffering, sorrow, pain, dissatisfaction.

There are different pleasures and some have tried to classify them. Thus, for example, Epicurus distinguishes between natural and necessary pleasures, natural and non-necessary pleasures and non-natural and non-necessary pleasures. According to Kant, there are distinctions between pleasure of the pleasant, which refers to what is pleasant for the senses, pleasure of the beautiful, "disinterested" pleasure of contemplation or representation and pleasure of the good, which is related to morality.

3.1.2.   2. A connection with emotions and mood

To talk about pleasure, it is necessary to put it in the broader context of emotions: "Sudden and momentary affective reaction, pleasant or painful, often accompanied by physical manifestations." "Constellation of responses of high intensity that include typical expressive, physiological and subjective manifestations".

What is the relationship between emotion and pleasure? If for some, pleasure is an emotion, it is generally considered, next to excitement, as a fundamental component of emotions.

One must also consider at once the fact that the emotions arrive on a bottom of mood. "This fundamental affective disposition, rich of all the emotional and instinctive instances, which give to each of our states of mind a pleasant or unpleasant tone, oscillating between the two extreme poles of pleasure and pain. The mood is to the thymic sphere which includes all the affections what is the conscience to the noetic sphere which includes all the representations, it is at the same time the most elementary and the most general manifestation. The basis of the affective life is made of a scale of moods as the basis of the representative life of a scale of consciousnesses."

Emotions are generally considered to be more abrupt, intense and transient, and mood as a background variable, more stable. The "hedonic tone" exists in two aspects, emotion and mood, corresponding to the variables of the hedonic "dashboard".[32]

3.2. 2. The process

3.2.1.   .1. The links between pleasure and motivation

Pleasure accompanies an action or a situation, but it also acts as a positive incentive to action. This idea implies that of reward and conditioning which we will develop in the chapter on addictions.

Emotion, motivation, reinforcement and arousal are related and often discussed together when discussing pleasure. Focusing on survival functions and circuits, these different elements can be seen as components of a single process that unfolds when an organism is faced with a challenge or opportunity.[33] The simplest pleasures appear to be useful for the survival of the individual and the species: the pleasure of drinking, eating, and sexual pleasure are the most obvious, but one could extend this idea and find such an "ancestral" core around which many other pleasures are built.

Pleasure plays a role in the adaptation of behavior for physiological purposes and therefore varies according to the state of the organism. The term alliesthesia has been proposed to describe the fact that the same stimulus can be perceived as pleasant or unpleasant depending on the internal state of the subject who receives it.[34]

Temperature, food, survival, the examples presented are at a fundamental level, they involve basic needs, but the search for satisfaction can also be guided by the presence of psychological needs. One will seek to satisfy these needs, to reach a more complex balance and one will be able to draw pleasure from it.

3.2.2. .2 Neurobiology

Regarding neurobiological studies, several things need to be clarified. First, it is important to emphasize the differences between "liking" and "wanting". There are partly different brain mechanisms responsible for these two aspects. Second, the circuits underlying basic pleasures, such as food-related pleasures and more elaborate pleasures, largely overlap.

Hotspots have been discovered. When stimulated, they increase the liking reactions of rodents to stimuli such as the sweetness of sugar.[35][36]

These are located at the level of the nucleus accumbens shell, and the ventral pallidum but also at the level of the bridge and at the cortical level (orbito-frontal cortex).

There are several things to note about these centers. Firstly, the reactions vary according to the type of substance injected into them. Second, there are centers that decrease liking reactions ("coldspots") and a certain number of them are also located in the shell of the nucleus accumbens, forming a kind of keyboard, a hedonic gradient. Thirdly, the "wanting" reactions can be dissociated from the pleasure reactions.[37] In particular, the role of dopamine, which plays a central role in motivation, would not have the same role in the generation of pleasure.

The role of the cortex is important in the neurobiology of pleasure, which is reflected in neuroimaging by an activity of the orbitofrontal cortex which follows the subjective feeling of pleasure and which decreases with satiety. [38] There seems to be a gradient from lateral to medial in the direction of pleasure, combined with another gradient from posterior to anterior in the direction of a greater abstraction of this pleasure. However, this activity would mainly reflect an involvement in the anticipation, evaluation and use of this type of stimuli rather than a generation of pleasure *per se.*

The orbitofrontal cortex thus has an important role in the neurobiology of pleasure.[39] However, medical observations (e.g. a history of severe herpes encephalopathy) show that pleasure as such can occur without these cortical regions.[40]

More generally, hotspots are integrated into circuits such as the reward circuit (to which we will return) which themselves interact with other circuits corresponding to cognitive, social and moral functions.

3.2.3. .3 Psychoanalysis: the pleasure principle and the relationship between pleasure and excitation

We will simply define the pleasure principle and use it as a starting point to evoke ideas about the relationship between pleasure and excitement. In the psychoanalysis part of the dictionary of philosophy we find: "Mode of perception analogous to sensations, but concerning internal stimuli, the pleasure-displeasure scale corresponds, according to Fechner, to the relative states of stability and instability of the organism. Taking up the notion, Freud simplifies it, by assimilating pleasure and discharge of excitation, and he raises it to the rank of an economic principle tending to reduce excitations to zero."

In the "vocabulary of psychoanalysis"[13] of Jean Laplanche and J-B

Pontalis states: "Pleasure principle: One of the two principles governing, according to Freud, mental functioning: the whole of psychic activity is aimed at avoiding displeasure and procuring pleasure. Insofar as displeasure is linked to the increase of the quantities of excitation and pleasure to their reduction, the pleasure principle is an economic principle."

In the rest of the article, we evoke the other great principle, the principle of reality, which interacts with the principle of pleasure: "The impulses would first seek only to be discharged, to be satisfied by the shortest ways. They would gradually learn about reality which alone allows them, through the necessary detours and postponements, to reach the sought-after satisfaction.

Freud's ideas are part of a series of theories that present the reduction of a variable such as arousal as a goal for individuals, but other models are proposed. For example, in Apter's model, arousal can be interpreted by an organism in two different ways as follows.

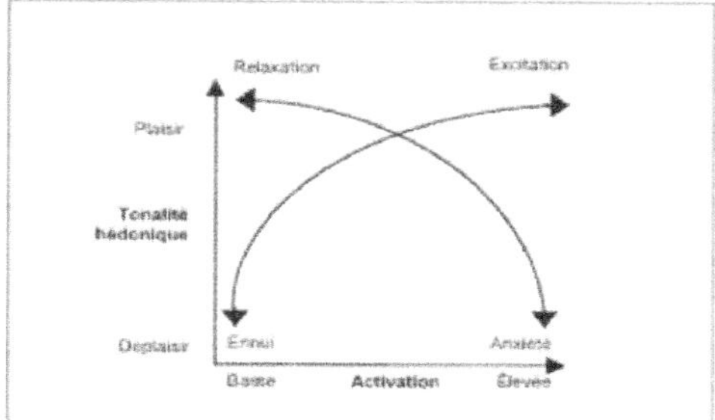

Figure 1: Apter's reversal theory

It should be noted that a reversal can occur, causing the passage from one curve to the other. It also introduces the notion of telic and paratelic modes. These are two meta-motivational modes, corresponding to the two curves of the diagram. The telic mode corresponds to the flight from excitement and has as its main characteristic the orientation towards a goal, towards the future, the spirit of seriousness; the paratelic mode corresponds to the search for excitement, it is oriented towards activity, the present moment, immediate amusement. These modes are used alternately by individuals; the same situation can therefore be apprehended by the same person in two different modes, even if statistically an individual will have a tendency to be in this or that mode.

The causes of reversal from one mode to the other can be divided into three classes: contingent events (the largest and most diverse class); frustrations in the search for satisfaction in one of the modes; satiety (the dynamic accompanying an event or activity and driving the reversal).[41]

3.3. 3. Man facing his pleasure

"Happiness, the most beautiful and best of things is also the most pleasant"

We have discussed the links between pleasure and motivation; we have seen how pleasure can on the one hand accompany and on the other hand lead us to the satisfaction of a need or to the restoration of a balance; we have evoked the hypothesis of its origin in a system which at the beginning is useful to our survival. These explanations can give the illusion that Man follows a hedonistic instinct and that he is the plaything of a process that he undergoes. Plunged into a world that exceeds him, Man finds himself confronted with his emotions, suffering, pleasure, he questions himself and tries to take a stand. He composes with these phenomena to build his existence as much as those build it.

In this perspective, the problem of the value of pleasure arises. To what extent should we listen to it, seek it out, distrust it? This problem is very old; almost all philosophers have tackled the subject, so we will not go into the details of the different doctrines.

This question about the value of pleasure cannot be understood without a deeper questioning. What is a happy life, full of meaning, worth living? Each of us constructs answers to these questions, answers that evolve as our experiences accumulate, as our environment changes, as we move forward in life. The value we give to pleasure "in itself" may thus vary, but above all, the pleasure we get from a given action (or situation) will vary: it will depend on the meaning of the action in a broader context and on its compatibility with other values.

We have seen that pleasure guides us instinctively, but that we can try to free ourselves from this instinct to question the relationships

that it maintains with other aspirations. Pleasure is central to our lives, it is the subject of many questions and to conclude, here is Spinoza's advice on this subject.

"And it is certainly only a wild and sad superstition that forbids taking pleasure. For why is it better to appease hunger and thirst than to drive away melancholy? This is my argument and my conviction. No deity, nor anyone else but the envious, takes pleasure in my helplessness and sorrow, nor does he hold tears, sobs, fear, etc., which are signs of a helpless soul, to be virtue. On the contrary, the more we are affected by a greater joy, the more we pass to a greater perfection, that is, the more necessary it is that we participate in the divine nature. Therefore, to use things and to take pleasure in them as much as possible (not to the point of disgust, for that is no longer taking pleasure in them) is of a wise man. It is of a wise man, I say, to comfort himself and to repair his strength through pleasant food and drink taken in moderation, and also through perfumes, the charm of green plants, finery, music, gymnasium games, spectacles, etc., which everyone can use without harming others. The human body, in fact, is composed of a great number of parts of different nature, which are continually in need of new and varied nourishment, so that the body as a whole may be equally fit for all that may follow from its nature [...].Therefore this order of life is perfectly in accord both with our principles and with common practice; so that if there are other ways of living, this one is, in any case, the best and most recommendable."

3.4. 4. The environment

For each of the ideas presented in this chapter on pleasure, the environment has a role to play. Most of the stimuli that trigger emotion and pleasure come from it. The state of the organism is the product of its interaction with the environment, which will therefore have an impact on the phenomenon of alliesthesia. The environment has an impact on the distribution of "hotspots" in our brain.[43]

Pleasure has a central place in learning phenomena. Rewards and punishments are widely used to educate children and subsequently, society asserts laws and uses this principle: what is bad for society is punished, what is good is rewarded.

So pleasure and pain make us learn, but on the other hand we know that pleasure is learned. This is highlighted in Becker's study[44] which shows the sequence of changes in experiences and attitudes that lead someone to use marijuana for pleasure. Pleasure is socially constructed like that taken from eating oysters or drinking Campari. This process occurs through interaction with more experienced people who minimize the negative effects and draw attention to the positive aspects.

4. Addictions

IV.1 General

IV.1.1. Definitions

Addictions

The term addiction is commonly used in French. In the Larousse dictionary 2015, we are referred to "addictive conduct": "repetitive behavior more or less incoercible and harmful to health". This is a borrowing from English, the term is used for the first time in literature by Shakespeare in Henry V, but the term itself comes from the Low Latin "addictus" abandoned. In medieval law, the derivative "addictio" exists for a "constraint by body of a defaulting debtor".

In medicine, Goodman's definition is most often used: "The process by which a behavior, which may allow both the production of pleasure and escape from a feeling of internal discomfort, is employed in a manner characterized by the repeated impossibility of controlling that behavior (powerlessness) and its continuation despite the knowledge of its negative consequences (unmanageability)."

We also talk about addictive practices (as we do about sexual practices or sports practices), which has the advantage of focusing on substance *use behaviors* and integrating social determinants.

The concept of addiction without drugs is being affirmed. In the DSM 5, pathological gambling has been moved from the chapter on impulse control disorders to that on addictive disorders.

The distinction between use - abuse / harmful use - dependence

Use in itself is not a pathology. We must distinguish between risky use, situational risk (driving, pregnancy...) or quantitative risk.

Abuse and harmful use correspond to the realization of the risk. It then gives rise to "somatic, psycho-affective or social damage" (ICD 10)

Addiction is classically divided into psychological and physical dependence. It must be emphasized that psychological dependence is the consequence of a neurobiological brain dysfunction, and that it is therefore not the part of dependence that is the result of simple willpower. It corresponds to the need to find the pleasure produced by the substance or to avoid the psychological discomfort that occurs in its absence. It is essentially expressed by "craving", a compulsive search for the substance against reason and will, an expression of a major and uncontrollable need. Physical dependence corresponds to the need to consume in order to avoid withdrawal symptoms (all of the symptoms that appear in the event of withdrawal) and to the appearance of tolerance.

A.   Inappropriate use of a substance leading to clinically significant impairment or distress

B.   Manifested by at least 2 of the following signs occurring within a one-year period:

1. The substance is often taken in larger amounts and for a longer period of time than intended.

2. There is a persistent desire or unsuccessful attempts to stop or control substance use.

3. A lot of time is spent procuring the substance, consuming it or recovering from its effects.

4. Existence of a craving, strong desire or impulse to use. (Most often occurs in an environment in which the drug was usually obtained or used)

5. Repeated use of the substance results in the inability to fulfill major obligations at work, school, or home (e.g., repeated absences or poor performance at work related to substance use; repeated substance-related absences, suspensions, or exclusion from school; neglect of children or household).

6. Substance use is continued despite persistent or recurrent social or interpersonal problems caused or aggravated by the effects of the substance

7. Important social, work or leisure activities are stopped or reduced because of substance use.

8. Repeated use of the substance in situations in which it is physically dangerous (e.g. driving a car or operating machinery despite impairment by the substance).

9. Use of the substance is continued despite the existence of persistent or recurrent physical or psychological problems likely caused or aggravated by the substance.

10. Tolerance, defined by any of the following signs:

a.   Need to significantly increase the amount of substance to achieve the desired intoxication or effects.

b.   Significantly reduced effect with continued use of the same amounts of substance.

11. Withdrawal manifested by any of the following signs:

a.   Withdrawal syndrome characteristic of the substance.

b.   The same substance (or a closely related substance) is used to relieve or avoid withdrawal symptoms

Tableau 1: DSM 5 diagnostic criteria

The DSM 5

In the fifth and most recent version of the Diagnostic and Statistical Manual of Mental Disorders, the general framework is entitled "substance related disorders" and includes "substance use disorders" and "substance induced disorders". Compared to the previous version, the intermediate categories of risky use, abuse or harmful use disappear and are replaced by a single diagnosis. The criteria of the DSM 4 sub-categories have been merged, "craving" has been added and legal consequences no longer appear. These criteria are shown in Table 1. There are eleven of them and they are of four types: control problems (1-4), social problems (5-7), risky use (8-9) and pharmacological criteria (10-11). Only two criteria are sufficient. A gradation of the disorder appears with mild (2-3), moderate (4-5) and severe (6 or more) levels.

IV.1.2. Epidemiology

Since 1993, there has been a public interest group in France: the French Observatory of Drugs and Drug Addiction. On its website (http://www.ofdt.fr) it presents a large amount of epidemiological and statistical data, for example those of ILIAD (Local Indicators for Information on Addictions). There is a similar organization in Europe, here is its website, also very complete: http://www.emcdda.europa.eu.

In Europe, current trends show a decline in the number of heroin admissions for treatment, HIV infections linked to drug use, and deaths by overdose. This trend must be qualified on the one hand by epidemic outbreaks among users in Greece and

Romania (linked to a decline in harm reduction policies) and on the other hand by the appearance and development of synthetic opioids.

The new drug market is increasingly dynamic, global and innovative. Stimulants users easily switch from one product to another depending on the supply, historical opiate producers produce cannabis or cocaine... There are also new types of stimulants, in particular synthetic cathiones (e.g. mephedrone), synthetic cannabinoids. The development of an online market is also a trend to be highlighted.

IV.1.3. Different substances

There are a variety of terms used in French, which cover the products concerned by addictions. *Substances* or *products, psychotropic* or *psychoactive*. The term *drug*, although still used by some to designate any substance that is pharmacologically active on the body, most often refers to an illegal substance and the phenomenon of dependence.

Although the "product" approach is currently being abandoned in favor of a more global approach, it is useful to distinguish between different substances with their own characteristics (acute or chronic effects, risks, modes of consumption, history or social contexts), but also the type of consumption and the mode of administration.

In the latest version of the DSM 5, substances are classified into ten categories as shown in the following table.

Alcohol
Caffeine
Cannabis
Hallucinogens (classified as phencyclydine (PCP) and others)
Inhalants
Opioids
Sedatives - Hypnotics - Anxiolytics
Stimulants
Tobacco

Other (including many drugs, anabolic steroids, betel...)

Tableau 2: DSM 5 substance categories

IV.2 The processes

IV.2.1. The reinforcement and its sources

conditioning and reinforcement

Addictive objects can, from a psychological and neurobiological point of view, be considered as "rewards". An object or an event qualified as a reward is defined by three aspects: its capacity to induce a subjective feeling of pleasure (the hedonic aspect), its ability to arouse the desire and the search for such stimuli (motivation), its positive impact on learning (reinforcement).[45] Addictions can be seen as a disruption of this reward system, as a "deregulation of hedonic homeostasis".

We can distinguish two types of reinforcement: positive reinforcement: the substances bring pleasure, which encourages people to try again; and negative reinforcement: the substances allow people to get out of a distressing situation, and in particular the withdrawal syndrome, which encourages them to try again when a distressing situation arises.

The opposing processes

The theory of opposing processes[46] , illustrated below, maintains that there is a stereotyped affective dynamic: positive or negative peak, adaptation to a lower level, plateau, end of stimulation, reverse peak, adaptation, plateau, return to normal.

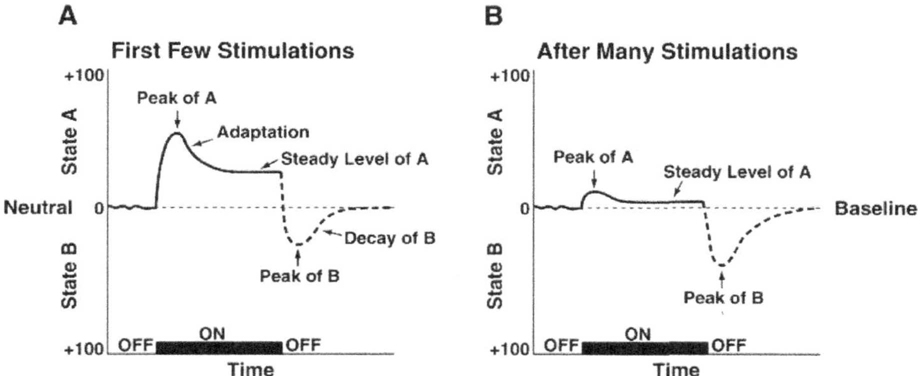

Figure 2: Opposing processes and evolution after numerous stimulations

It can be applied to addictions: with time, the positive peak diminishes, the withdrawal syndrome and the negative emotions become more important, and the subject will tend to use the substance that was responsible for the positive reaction to restore the hedonic balance.

Incentive awareness

Another theory is that of the sensitization of the incentive.[47] It postulates an adaptation of the nervous system, a sensitization of a system by certain substances, i.e. an ever-increasing effect of substances on this system. This effect is expressed both on the neurochemical and behavioral levels. The system in question is the one that attributes an incentive salience to actions, stimuli, their perceptions or mental representations.

Thus the substances that sensitize the circuit in question make themselves more and more wanted, more and more desired. This desire has a behavioral consequence and explains the "craving". This theory accounts for a dissociation between pleasure and wanting, between "liking" and "wanting". The changes in the nervous system are long-term changes, perhaps definitive, which explains the relapse phenomenon.

IV.2.2. Neurobiology

A distinction is often made between the different phases of addiction: intoxication, withdrawal and negative affect, and preoccupation and anticipation.[48,49] Figure 3 below summarizes the different phases and the structures involved. The mesocorticolimbic dopamine system has a central role in the processes of conditioning, reinforcement, learning, motivation and of course in addiction. It constitutes what can be called a reward circuit. [50] It seems that the positive reinforcement linked to the use of substances is largely mediated by an increase in dopamine in this system and in particular in the nucleus accubens.[50]

These increases in dopamine lead to a decrease in the number of D2 dopamine receptors in addicted users and a decrease in the amount released. These elements reflect a depression of the reward system and help explain a decrease in sensitivity to natural reinforcers. This decrease in sensitivity is also found in fMRI[51]

The theory of allostatic neuroadaptation sees in the chronic elevation of the reward threshold a central element in the development of addictions.[52] Gradually the sensations of pleasure diminish but the sensations of discomfort remain and a new equilibrium is established but at a lower level.

The preoccupation and anticipation stage is marked mainly by changes in the glutamatergic circuitry, connecting the medial part of the prefrontal cortex, the nucleus accumbens and the ventral pallidum.[49]

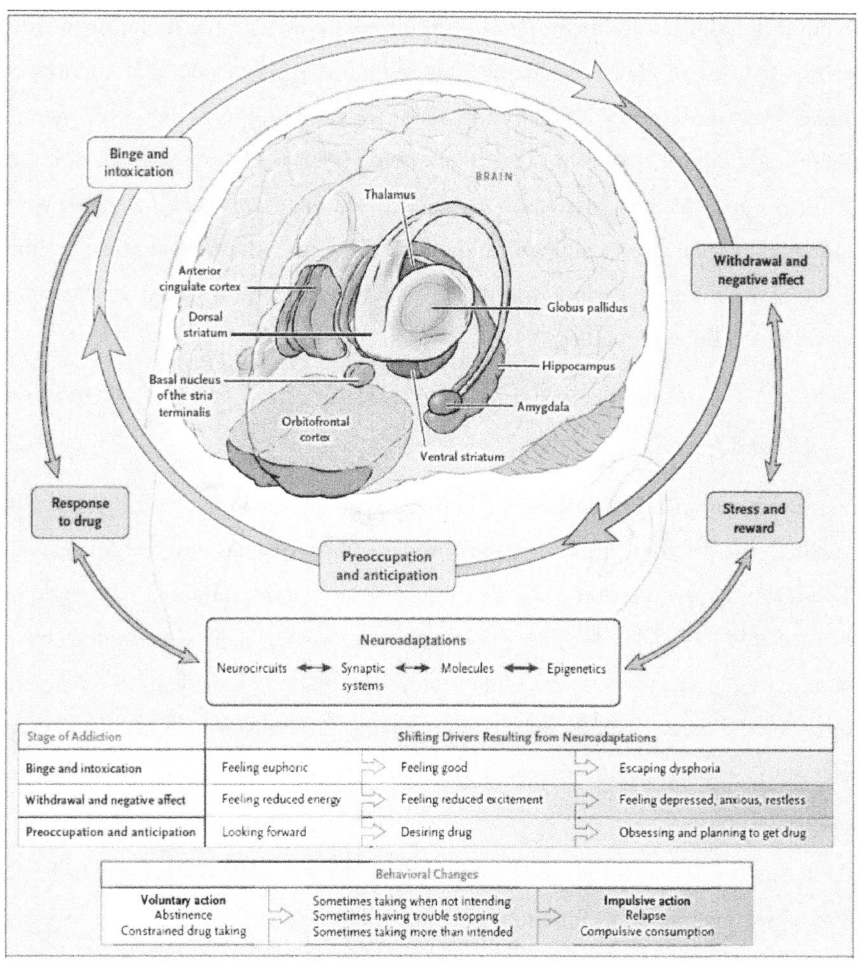

Stage of Addiction	Shifting Drivers Resulting from Neuroadaptations		
Binge and intoxication	Feeling euphoric	Feeling good	Escaping dysphoria
Withdrawal and negative affect	Feeling reduced energy	Feeling reduced excitement	Feeling depressed, anxious, restless
Preoccupation and anticipation	Looking forward	Desiring drug	Obsessing and planning to get drug

Behavioral Changes		
Voluntary action Abstinence Constrained drug taking	Sometimes taking when not intending Sometimes having trouble stopping Sometimes taking more than intended	**Impulsive action** Relapse Compulsive consumption

Figure 3: Different stages of the addiction cycle and brain structures involved. From "Neurobiologic Advances from the Brain Disease Model of Addiction[48]

Stress-related circuits are also put forward.[52] In the conjunction of stressful environmental events with other individual factors, this aspect has a particular importance upstream, in the construction of a vulnerability to addictions and a vulnerability to relapse. The hypothalamic-pituitary-adrenergic axis is activated in certain stressful situations and many brain structures, in particular the dopaminergic neurons which have glucocorticoid receptors, will be sensitive to these changes and will be durably modified by them. This last point is of considerable importance since it underlines the role of the environment. This last point is of considerable importance as it underlines the role of the environment. Indeed, in presenting the systems modified by addictions, we do not really talk about what leads one individual rather than another from use to addiction. The explanations are genetic, epigenetic, environmental, explanations supported by a number of adoption studies, animal models, exploring genes coding for receptors or enzymes, involved in neuronal transmission or cellular signalling.[53]

IV.2.3. *Psychoanalysis: narcissistic fragility, attachment disorders*

"The psychodynamic approach to addictions has gone from the objectal side distinguishing the different figures on the clinical and psychopathological levels (side for which it would be rather the effects of the conduct than its function that would be decisive for the subject), to their common narcissistic side determined by a disturbance of the processes of separation-individuation linked to a traumatic bankruptcy of the early environment, compromising the transitional and introjection processes until weakening the narcissistic bases, the self-esteem and the feeling of inner security.[54]

How does this behaviour allow the problem to be "resolved"? "The recourse to the addictive object supports a function of protection against the threat of psychic collapse, of annihilation linked to the insufficient differentiation of the maternal object: "it allows the addict's ego to obtain an immediate change of state, to find another subjective state, (...), that of the origins of the psychic apparatus", this psychic state of all creative power and independence that Rado qualified as "original narcissistic dimension of the Ego". This state can take the form of an ecstasy, a drunkenness or be simply a restoration of a sufficient interior security.[54]

J. Mac Dougall also mentions a deep and ancient potential cause of addictions. Because of her anxieties and unconscious fears and desires, a mother is potentially capable of creating an addictive relationship with her baby, both to her presence and to her care, by inhibiting the narcissistic value that her baby's mobility, alertness, intelligence, and sensitivity may have. "Thus, food, drugs, alcohol, tobacco, or others, can temporarily alleviate psychic stress and, in other words, fulfill a maternal function that the addicted person is unable to do for herself. These addictive objects then take the place of the transitional objects of childhood (and whose proper function is to incorporate the maternal environment), which at the same time should have freed the child from his or her bond of dependence on the mother."[55] The psychic stress in question can be of several kinds: neurotic anxiety, psychotic anxiety, depression, damaged narcissistic image.

IV.3. The people

We have seen the characteristics of addictive practices and their most recent diagnostic criteria. But why will an individual develop an addiction? Why this individual rather than another? To clarify this question, Dr. Olievenstein's phrase that "addiction" is the meeting of a product, a personality and a socio-cultural moment, has become classic. M. Reynaud gives us a less lyrical formula, but which goes in the same direction:

Addiction = P.I.E

P refers to product-related risk factors, I to individual vulnerability factors and E to environmental risk factors. Besides affective states (anxiety, depression) which play a major role, we have chosen to develop personality factors and psychiatric disorders.

IV.3.1. The personality

In the field of individual vulnerability factors, personality traits have their place. A high level of sensation seeking would be a vulnerability factor to all addictions; it corresponds to "the search for varied, new, complex and intense sensations and experiences, and by the willingness to take physical, social, legal and financial risks, to obtain such experiences."[56]

Low self-esteem, shyness, self-deprecation, excessive emotional reactions (or the opposite), difficulties in having stable relationships, in reacting to certain events or in solving interpersonal problems are highlighted[57] . Other authors add: a high level of novelty seeking[58] , a high level of emotional reactivity, a low level of danger avoidance, a slow return to equilibrium after stress, a high level of behavioral activities associated with low attentional capacities.

Alongside this dimensional approach, a categorical approach, although criticized, finds personality disorders varying according to the type of substance: a higher prevalence of antisocial personality for heroin, antisocial, narcissistic and borderline personality for cocaine. It should be noted that most people suffering from addiction do not have personality disorders and that there is not *one* but *many* different personalities.[59]

IV.3.2. Psychiatric disorders

The relationships between psychoactive substances, addictions, and psychiatric disorders are deep and complex. Without prejudging the order in which they appear, there are strong epidemiological links.[60,61]

The study of co-occurring psychiatric disorders is a fundamental step in the medical management of an addiction problem. The type of relationship can be summarized as follows:[62]

- Both disorders have an independent etiopathogeny. Their diagnosis, treatment and evolution can be considered individually

- Co-occurrence is due to iatrogenic causes

- The onset of mental disorders is a direct, psychotoxic effect of the consumption of the psychoactive substance

- There is a shared psychobiological vulnerability, developing a synergic interaction that generates the appearance of a new pathology with its own clinical picture.

- Mental disorders facilitate the development of addictions. We can apply the hypothesis of self-medication which maintains that the drugs used would improve the psychiatric pathology

Dual pathology" is the appearance in a patient with psychiatric disorders and addictions of synergistic processes between the two pathologies, leading to a modification of the symptoms, a decrease in the effectiveness of the treatments and the aggravation and chronicisation of their evolution.

IV.4. The environment

On an individual level and from birth, the environment can shape vulnerability factors (stressful environments, family factors...), and then provide triggering situations that combine with these factors to progress towards addiction. Social inequalities appear as a risk factor for additive practices in the "social causality" of addictions and conversely addictions influence social trajectories.

Social factors are obvious since substance use occurs in a social setting with a peer group. On a more cultural level, the environment is also important.[63] Cultural factors can be defined as the set of interpretations of the effects of a substance (or stimulation), which are specific to a given culture and which in turn influence the addictive potential of the substance (or stimulation). We can, for example, put into perspective the ravages of the massive introduction of opium into China in the 19th century, whereas its culturally integrated use in India did not pose a problem.

We will finish with a vision of the influence of the current society on the addictive problems: "Addiction, as suffering, excess, is one of the ways caused by the liberal society which constitutes a libidinal economy aiming at capturing the libido of the individuals in order to attract their investment on objects of the consumption generating profits. This type of exploitation of the libidinal economy is a fundamental characteristic of our post-modern society, in which consumption manifests itself as a claim to identity at both the individual and social levels. The "new malaise in civilization" to which certain current pathologies respond, and more particularly Addiction, is characterized by a valorization of this economy that destroys desire, insofar as it reduces the object of desire to an accessible object - and at the same time destroys it since the very nature of this object is to be infinite."[64]

5. Mutual influences

V.1 The Myth

Since antiquity, links between art and alcohol exist. They are embodied for example in the figure of Dionysus: god of wine and theater. The myth of the artist using psychoactive substances has crossed the centuries and is still present in the current society. Today, there are numerous newspaper and magazine articles, television programs and a large number of biographies and autobiographies of artists that use this approach.[65]

The book " The imaginary of drugs "[66] of Max Milner can enlighten us to understand these relations. For the author, the imaginary of drugs has a double meaning. Firstly that of imaginary produced by the drugs, that is to say "what the artists added to the field of the imaginary thanks to them".

We will address this question later by asking how these substances influence creativity?

The second meaning is: the imaginary related to drugs: the works dealing more or less incidentally with drugs, users and their psychology.

We can see that it is mainly the artists themselves, through their works, who have produced this myth. Thomas de Quincey is considered the initiator of this literary theme, with his "Confessions of an English Opium Eater", published in 1821. Following him, from the "Hashischins" club to the "beat generation", from painting to music, the theme of drugs has never ceased to be present in art, through works and artists.

The "imaginary relating to the drugs" is not limited to the produced works. It has a link with social and cultural conceptions, and in particular with "the bohemian life". The figure of the bohemian "is a form of social protest which, through a certain theatricalization, allows a putting at distance of the social world and its conventions, of the tensions generated by the relations that the individual maintains with its social destiny." This bohemian life is often translated by the use of alcohol, drugs, but the methods have evolved with time.

Thus, from the second half of the 20th century, we witness a change of scale: democratization of eccentricity, massification of bohemian life, change of the main vector from literature to music and the figure of the rock star gradually becoming the model of the artist's life.[67] Then from the 1990s, the very notion of bohemia and the representation of the links between drugs and artists changes: appearance of the figure of the bohemian bourgeois who becomes a new standard, development of techno music parties, electro, where the artist fades behind the collective, change of the social representations of the drug users...[67]

Even more recently, the figure of the "surviving artist" has developed, who has used drugs at some point in his or her creative career and who, with maturity, has found the path to redemption. Drug rehabs are nowadays a common part of the image of the artist's life and are often publicized.[67]

Thus the figure of the artist using psychoactive substances has evolved over the years. In this chapter, we will try to better understand if a link exists in reality and what can explain it.

V.2 The reality

In an attempt to overcome a popular belief, some studies have tried to examine the link between artistic creativity and substance use with a scientific method, to establish a statistical relationship. Published studies are quite rare, probably due to methodological limitations. As for the existence of a link, the results are not very clear. Moreover, the results are generally based more on problems of abuse and dependence than on use.

Andreasen[21] , which we have already mentioned, finds 30% of writers with alcohol problems (compared to 7% among controls), no difference for other drugs: 7% in both groups.

Kyaga[22] found an association only for writers: OR 1.47 (CI: 1.25-1.74) for alcohol and OR: 1.53 (CI: 1.09 - 2.16) for drugs. For other artistic activities the relationship is negative: not significant for alcohol (OR: 0.98, CI: 0.95 - 1.01), significant for other substances: OR: 0.84 (CI: 0.79 - 0.89) and very frankly negative for scientific occupations! (OR 0.34 and 0.25 for alcohol and other substances respectively).

A 2009 study[68] , is based on the responses of 431 members (327 women) of student fraternities to the *Adjective Check List* (personality test) and the *Core Alcohol and Drug Survey*. No association was found between creative personality and drug and alcohol use. An interesting point in this study is that people with creative personalities believe significantly more than others that alcohol makes them more creative.

If a link exists, what type of link is it?

One of the first to have asked the question, and to have tried to answer it in a rational way, is A. Ludwig who distinguishes 10 types of possible interaction between alcohol and creativity.[69] Alcohol can increase or decrease creativity, directly or indirectly. (4 types of relationships). Creativity can lead to a decrease or increase in alcohol consumption, directly or indirectly (4 other types). Alcohol and creativity may simply be present without any relationship to each other, and ultimately an intervening factor may alter alcohol consumption and creativity in either direction.

Once this typology is presented, he analyzes the biographies of 34 people who spent at least part of their lives in the $XX^{\text{ème}}$ century, selected on the basis of alcohol consumption (corresponding to the concept of alcohol dependence) and creative achievements (people who have seen at least one of their posthumous biographies published, and cited in the New York Times review of books since 1965). The total exceeds 100%, as the relationships may have changed during the author's lifetime: for 76.5% alcohol directly affected creativity, and for 17.6% indirectly. For only 8.8% alcohol was directly responsible for an increase in creativity, but for 50% it was indirectly responsible. Creativity was indirectly responsible for the increase in alcohol consumption for almost a third of those studied (32.4%) (5.8% directly). It was the cause of a decrease in consumption, directly for 11.8% and indirectly for only one person, i.e. 2.9%. A third factor modifying both alcohol intake and creativity was found in 38.2% of the artists studied, and finally the two were independent for 44.1%.

These percentages do not have any real statistical significance, but they do give trends and, above all, underline the complexity of the relationship between psychoactive substances and creation. We will not use these 10 categories as they are, but we will draw inspiration from them.

Firstly, the two entities, psychoactive substances and creation, can influence each other, directly or indirectly. The two following parts have as main objective to understand what pushes creators, artists, to use psychoactive products. We will thus speak essentially about the effects of mutual increase, the effects of drive. Secondly, the two entities can have common causes, have their place in similar processes, which explains their proximity. We will develop this idea in the last two parts.

V.3. Art under influence ?

An artist meets a product that will have pharmacological effects on him. This substance will modify his state of consciousness, his perceptions, his concentration, his mood... These modifications depend on the type of product, the individual, the context... many parameters. The first hypothesis is that the artist will more or less consciously use these modifications, these alterations, these exogenous influences, for his work. We will thus see in a first time how these substances (in particular alcohol, which is the most studied), can be used to start, support, modify, or finally interrupt the creative process.

In the rest of the chapter, we will move away from the core of the creative process to focus on the person and his or her environment. We will insist on the fact, reported in several studies, that an anticipatory effect, independent of the pharmacological effect, takes place and influences the creator.

To approach the direct pharmacological effect, and for a question of condition of experimentation, we will initially focus on the creative act as if it had a beginning, a middle and an end. However, in practice, artists feed their whole life with experiences, sensations, encounters, which they will use in their work, which will influence them. The impact of the substances can be felt in this "exploratory" phase, as long and diffuse as it is, without the work being directly elaborated under the influence of the product. This is what we will discuss at the end of this section.

V.3.1. A direct influence?

Our understanding of the creative process is fragmentary. Although they can be grouped into different families, each psychoactive substance, on each individual, has different cognitive and emotional effects. It therefore seems illusory to claim to explain in detail the direct effect of drugs on the creative process. We will simply try to show that it is possible that some effects exist and can possibly be sought by certain artists.

Our first source of information comes of course from the artists themselves, but faced with cognitive effects which remain rather vague - we speak of visions, of inspiration - researchers have tried to measure, by scientific methods, the said effects. The few studies we present here are not exhaustive and concern mainly alcohol and cannabis, the most studied substances. It is likely that studies on cocaine or other stimulants will find different effects (on the maintenance of concentration, the capacity to work, the elaboration phase more than the inspiration phase).

With respect to alcohol

The associations of ideas seem to be more numerous but of lesser quality and less objective. For Nash (1962), a low dose (blood concentration < 0.09%) seemed to improve verbal abilities. With a design that allowed drinking on demand (Hajcak 1976), originality was improved, but fluency and creative problem-solving ability (RAT) were lowered. In another study (Koski-Jannes 1983), the total number of ideas was improved, but their quality was reduced. Finally, some studies found no effect of alcohol at low doses.[70]

A 1965 study[71], studied the responses to the Thematic Apperception Test (TAT) (4 images per story, a story to be invented from them, and this on 3 occasions) of students in natural conditions (discussion in a living room or party), according to their alcohol consumption. She found effects according to the number of drinks: progressive increase of ideas of physical aggression, then of physical sex, then decrease of restrictions of aggression, fear, anxiety, sensitivity to time.

Another study dating from 1974[72] , studied 49 women between 21 and 32 years old. This study is forty years old and it can be noted that at the time men also participated (without being the object of the study), to "avoid that women drink in a female-only environment, which is unusual and would not have seemed natural to them"! The TATs consisted of 5 images and were administered before and 70 minutes after the party began. Femininity seemed to increase and ideas of power decreased.

In a 1989 study conducted by Gustafson[73] , 60 Swedish students were divided into three groups: alcohol (Vodka and tonic), placebo and control. They had to perform a Rotter test to determine the internal/external level of their locus of control and a Gestalt Completion Test of Street, after drinking. For the locus of control, alcohol made the subjects significantly less "internal" (i.e., they attributed the events that affected them more to external circumstances than to their own actions). The Gestalt Completion Test was evaluated according to their "distance to the stimulus". The results showed that the responses of the "alcohol" group were less close to the stimulus. A very similar study[74] but for women, with 60 female students, found similar results.

The result of the latter three studies can be interpreted as a relative reinforcement of the primary process by alcohol.

Norlander and Gustafson conducted a series of five studies, each corresponding to a phase of the creative process described by Wallas. For the preparatory phase[75] 42 people completed tests of deductive reasoning (syllogisms) and persistent effort, while divided into three groups: "alcohol" (at 1 mL of 100% alcohol/kg), "placebo" or "control". The "alcohol" and "placebo" groups performed worse on the persistent effort test and the "alcohol" group performed worse on the deductive reasoning test.

For the incubation[76] , 60 participants were divided into three groups using the model and doses of the previous study. All sober, they had to plan aloud an experiment examining the relative parts of heredity and environment. Then they went home and drank the prescribed dose of alcohol or placebo. The next day they had to take notes on the subject in a notebook provided, then drink the same dose again before going to bed, and finally write a final report. While the scientific value did not vary, the results of the incubation phase in the alcohol group notebooks were more extensive and their final reports more original.

For the illumination phase[77] , 21 members of the authors' society and 21 controls were each divided into three groups according to the same design as in the previous studies, i.e., 6 groups. The creativity test consisted of giving possible uses for objects. The answers were analyzed by 2x2 judges. The results showed: that the alcohol group had less flexibility, more originality, and that there was no difference between the authors and the non-authors.

Finally for the verification phase[78] : 42 students, 21 men, 21 women, divided in the three usual groups, had to read the poem "Vid Hashorna", by the Swedish author Erik Axel Karlfeld (poem chosen for the large amount of images it contains). All participants, after reading the poem, had to make a sketch illustrating it. Then each participant received his or her glass and was instructed to transform the sketch into a finished drawing, using colored pencils only. 2X3 judges evaluated the final products for both originality and handicraft quality. The different groups did not show any difference in originality but the alcohol group was less good on the technical side.

For the authors, the conclusion of this series of studies is that a moderate amount of alcohol hinders the phases of creation that are mainly based on the secondary process: preparation, verification and some phases of illumination; but facilitates those mainly based on the primary process: incubation, some phases of illumination and restitution (or recovery).

With regard to cannabis

Few studies examine the effects of cannabis on creativity. Block's[79] focuses on the acute cognitive effects of cannabis use (as well as differences related to inhalation time). 48 adults between the ages of 18 and 42 were asked to puff on a 19 mg Δ^9 -THC marijuana cigarette every 35 seconds, or on a placebo (THC-free marijuana) cigarette. A series of cognitive tests were performed: psychomotor, concept formation, free or constrained associations, text learning, pair learning, Buschke's test (list learning, cueing and uncueing), a short test of academic ability and the Iowa Test of Educational

Development", including questions on vocabulary, arithmetic... All abilities were reduced under cannabis except two: vocabulary tests and concept formation. More interesting in our case, associations (freely associating a word with a given word, or associating a word with a constraint such as being in the same category, being a property, being opposite to the word) are slower but more original, less common.

The study conducted by V. Curran[80] in 2002, like the previous study, explored against placebo the effects of cannabis on several cognitive tests: memory, logic... in 15 participants. This time it was ingested, in the form of a 15 or 7.5 mg capsule of Δ^9 -THO. Some tests were unchanged (logic, working memory), the bulk of the tests were disturbed, but at 6 h verbal fluency (for the highest dose) was improved, which might be in the direction of disinhibition of information retrieval in semantic memory.

Regarding hallucinogens

Besides alcohol and cannabis, a small part of the literature focuses on hallucinogenic substances. O. Janiger then B. Sessa[81] give us reviews several decades apart that have served as guides.

In 1955, Berlin studied the effects of mescaline (400-700 mg) and LSD (50 µg) on 4 graphic artists. While technical execution deteriorated, a panel of experts judged the work of "greater aesthetic value" than their usual work.

In 1963, F. Barron administered psilocybin to a number of highly creative individuals and collected their impressions. He concluded that "psilocybin dissolves many definitions, melts boundaries, and allows experiences of greater intensity or extreme value to take place, in many dimensions.

Mc Glothlin, in 1967, had 72 students perform a battery of creativity tests before and one week after taking 200 µg of LSD. 62% had a better appreciation of music in the post LSD period. They bought more records, visited more museums, and went to listen to music more often, without any objectified increase in their sensitivity or creative performance.

Zegans in 1967, studied the effects of 0.5 µg/kg of LSD on the creativity tests of 19 volunteers, 11 receiving a placebo. The results are not statistically significant, but a tendency seems to exist in favour of a greater creativity under LSD, in particular in individuals with a "creative personality".

Finally a study conducted by J.W. Fadiman and W.W Harmann in 1966, studied the effects of 200 µg of mescaline in 27 individuals engaged in professions requiring creative abilities (mathematicians, physicists, architects...). The environment was favorable and the

participants conditioned to feel a benefit. The tests showed better results on mescaline, and the subjective effects were positive. 50% felt a net benefit, 30% had difficulty concentrating during the session, and 20% were somewhere in between.

O. Janiger's study and its history are interesting.[82] It began in the spring of 1955. During this study, a total of 2000 doses of 2.5 µg/kg of LSD were administered to 848 people (including Carry Grant), and their impressions collected. 2 types of environment were possible: a comfortable living room or an artist's studio with the necessary equipment for painting, sculpting, drawing, and access to an adjoining garden.

The art sub-project began serendipitously when one of the first participants, a professional artist, picked up a "Kachina" deer (dolls representing New Mexican and Arizona Indian spirits) during the experiment and drew it furiously, exclaiming afterwards, "This is like four years of art school!"

Over a period of seven years, 70 active professional artists participated, 20 of whom produced a before and after LSD series of 56 "Kachina" deer. Their work was analyzed by a California art professor in eight aspects.

The main changes were in the general style (more expressionist, less objective), the intensification of color and texture, the lines (more flowing or angular), and the broadening of the composition. The author does not comment on the relative value of the works, but emphasizes that subjectively, for the artists, these works were more interesting, and that the psychedelic experience produced positive and lasting effects on their work, influenced their artistic development, and may have represented a creative crisis to reach another level of expression.

To summarize, the results of these hallucinogen studies do not clearly show a net benefit for creativity tests, but overwhelmingly report a subjective and lasting improvement for the artists.

To conclude on the *direct influences,* "comprehensive" hypotheses have been put forward. The most coherent one seems to us to be disinhibition[83,84] . One seeks to bring to the surface associations, combinations, which would be judged irrelevant, if one were to function in an analytical, systematic way. It is the kind of effect sought during the reveries of the solitary walker. An abundance of associations, comparisons, construction of ideas, more or less coherent or adapted, takes place in an "automatic", "unconscious" way. Certain psychoactive substances could not only encourage this process, but above all lift, at least in part, its inhibition, its control. According to Knafo[85] it is a regressive process that is at work.

Carson[83] proposes a more complete model of vulnerability factors shared between creativity and psychopathology and in particular between creativity and alcoholism. A lowered latent inhibition, i.e. the incapacity to exclude, to filter certain stimuli, is a common factor of vulnerability to drug taking and creativity. Alongside this latent inhibition, sensation seeking and neural hyperconnectivity are vulnerability factors. Protective factors: high IQ, developed working memory and high cognitive flexibility, interact with vulnerability factors to increase creativity.

A special focus should be placed on mood and emotions. Psychoactive substances can alter mood. Studies suggest that joy is associated with improved creative performance, and others suggest that sadness is as well. Thus emotions would facilitate creation. Several hypotheses have been put forward: emotions could put the individual in a mental state conducive to creation, others suggest that emotional experiences would be a means of associating ideas that are cognitively distant but emotionally close.

It is in bipolar disorders that this idea crystallizes. The links between this type of pathology and artistic creation are complex, the scientific literature is abundant on this subject and we have already touched on it in a section devoted to the links between psychiatric disorders and creativity. The important point to remember is that psychoactive substances can influence artists and their work by altering their mood and emotions.

V.3.2. An indirect influence?

Most of the testimonies and the studies quoted above, agree on the fact that the creative process is not fundamentally modified by drugs. It seems at best facilitated, uninhibited. Gilles Deleuze goes in this direction when he says: "[...] we realize more and more that where we thought alcohol or drugs were necessary, they are absolutely not necessary. Perhaps it is necessary to have gone through this to realize that everything we thought we could do thanks to it, to alcohol, we could do without it"[86]. If one can do without the drug to achieve the same result, the drug allows a control of the process. More than a modification, it is used to initiate, support or interrupt the creation.

Start

Many testimonies or case studies suggest that in art, the effect of drugs is indirect. It takes a certain amount of courage to start, to enter the creative process. The page or the blank canvas is often frightening, a room full of spectators can also be frightening for the actor or the musician. More than a direct cognitive impact, it is a start, an encouragement which is then evoked.

In her review, Day[87] tells us, "Alcohol can have a triggering role, can help overcome the anxiety of the blank page, what Simenon called stage fright, doubts about their ability to write, the quality of their work."

We can guess in Simenon's words, the stimulating effect, of support, that alcohol can have: "I started very early in the morning, at six o'clock in a general way, and I finished at the end of the afternoon; that represented two bottles, and eighty pages... I worked very fast, sometimes I wrote eight stories in one day".

In addition to alcohol, he could have recourse to Belladenal: "To overcome stage fright, to reassure himself, a tranquilizer tablet in his shirt pocket. Because the act of writing is, for him, dominated by fear. Writing is the shirt soaked in sweat, the fear of the blank page, of blocking, the fear of staying dry."[88]

In the article "alcohol input, creative output"[69] that we have already quoted, Ludwig gives us a similar example, quoting the American author E. B. White: "Before I start writing, I always treat myself to a nice dry Martini. Just one, to give me the courage to write. After that, I'm on my own."

These testimonies evoke less the ecstatic dream than the fuel to start and maintain the creation. This is also at times the point of view of P. Brenot[89] who tells us: " [...] toxic paradises will be a facilitating, activating or revealing intermediary of this daily exercise that creation requires, because we know how much anguish the blank page brings, how much "white paper, ink, the pen frighten me," said Cocteau, "I know that they are ganging up on my will to write", and how many creators will use artifice to continue their daily work.

A little further on in the same book: "If I had to add a virtue, to specify the necessity of the use of toxic substances so frequent among creators, I would insist on the "starter" effect that psychotropic drugs can have on the creative process and that has made their use so frequent. And he quotes Philippe Sollers on the subject of amphetamines: "They allow you to write faster. The warm-up time goes from one hour to ten minutes. The output is better. And this does not alter concentration and lucidity. [...] They produce an acceleration effect, allow faster associations of ideas and words, lift inhibitions..."

Stop

Once launched into a demanding, trying process, drugs, especially their sedative effects, can be used to turn the page, to relax, to escape from compulsive work and to return to it later, with new vitality. "Many authors have commented on their use of alcohol by explaining that it allowed them to relax after an intense period of work. Ernest Hemingway had a routine, according to which he got up early, wrote in the morning, fished or hunted in the afternoon, and drank at night to relax and decompress. He and William Faulkner explained that they drank to help them stop writing, to switch off the creative process.[87] Tolson agrees: "Winicks' survey of jazzmen and drugs indicates that drugs can be used to relax after five or six hours of playing emotionally demanding music.[90]

V.3.3. A role for the artist's expectations?

"I wanted to mend my ways with chocolate; I took some the day before yesterday to digest my dinner, in order to have a good supper, and I took some yesterday to nourish myself, in order to fast until the evening: it did all the things I wanted; this is why I find it pleasant, it is that it acts according to the intention" (October 28, 1671) Madame de Sévigné [91]

The effects of psychoactive substances depend of course on the substance itself, its molecular structure, the dose and the method of administration. But they also depend to a large extent on the expectations of the person using them. These effects find their translation in the placebo effect: the anticipation of a positive effect generates a positive effect, and this, outside of any psychotropic substance, of any pharmacological effect.

From this point of view, a study[92] from 1985 by A. Lang is very instructive. Underlining the lack of theoretical basis and the methodological shortcomings of previous studies, it is primarily exploratory and uses a "Balanced Placebo" design. 40 male students were randomly assigned to 4 groups: *thought they would receive alcohol/received alcohol, thought they would receive alcohol/not received alcohol, thought they would not receive alcohol/received alcohol and finally thought they would not receive alcohol/not received alcohol.* A number of pieces of information were collected before, during and after the creativity test, which consisted of a Torrance test.

The sample was almost equally divided between those who thought alcohol would help them and those who thought it would hurt them (45% - 55%). There was no alcohol-related difference in performance, but those who thought they had received alcohol rated their own work higher, and the only variable they thought explained this "success" was luck. Neither prior expectations nor mood had any statistical influence.

The author analyzes these results as follows: when they think they have drunk, people apply more lenient standards to their evaluation. "Handicapped" by intoxication, they do not have to defend their product as a reflection of their true ability. Such changes allow for a freedom from perfectionism and a reliance on instinct, in the sense that it facilitates initiation, maintenance, and enjoyment in the creative process.

In the study by Lapp, Collins and Izzo[93] , 116 men between 21 and 35 years of age had to reorganize in an "aesthetic" and "natural" way a set of 64 cards on which flowers of different shapes, sizes and numbers appeared. As in the previous study, a Placebo Design Scale was used. The authors carry out a rather complex analysis of the results, creativity being evaluated by the difference between the arrangement of the participants' cards and, on the one hand, a purely dimensional arrangement (i.e. based solely on the three characteristics of shape, number and color) and, on the other hand, a random arrangement. As in the previous study, no pharmacological effect was found, but this time a placebo effect was observed.

Another more recent study[94] hypothesizes that simple subtle cues, simple primers associated with alcohol or cannabis, will influence performance on the creativity test, depending on the subject's expectations.

The first of the two groups studied, for alcohol, involved 135 participants, and the second, for cannabis, 173. Before the creativity test itself, the participants had to solve a lexical decision test (to know if a string of characters briefly displayed corresponds to a word or not). Just before this string, words related to the substance under study were displayed for 40 ms (e.g., "beer" or "high"). The creativity test consisted of a Remote Associate Test. The subjects' expectations of the effect of the substances, their drug use and their mood were also assessed.

The results show that primers associated with substance use influence creative processes, in the sense that subjects expect the substance to influence them.

A second study (157 participants) presented in the same article used the same model, but only for alcohol, and added an arithmetic test. The results for the Alternate Use Test were consistent with the previous study, but not for the arithmetic test, which contradicts the hypothesis that primers generally increase attention.

These studies do not resolve all the questions they raise, not all the leads are in line, but it seems that consumer expectations play a significant role.

V.3.4. A source of inspiration?

The studies presented at the beginning of this section provide us with information about a possible direct or indirect impact on the creative process. A definition as precise as possible and the measurement of parameters are inevitable to advance in the understanding of our subject, but there are things that seem more difficult to quantify and the ideas presented here are not supported by scientific studies.

A rather small proportion of works have been realized directly under influence, and it is then in general about very particular conditions. For example, in the graphic arts, these are rapid techniques (drawing, watercolor...). This link with the speed of creation is also evoked by Fitzgerald when he says that he writes short stories because it lasts him a bottle, and that beyond that, to write a novel, it is no longer possible.

Most poets and writers influenced by drugs have written or rewritten extensively after using drugs. "Opium allows us to give form to the formless; it prevents us, alas, from communicating this privilege to others. Even if I lose sleep, I will watch for the unique moment of detoxification when this faculty will still function a little, inadvertently, with the return of communicative power."[95]

Day in his review of the literature agrees: "In reality very little work of quality appears to have been written under the direct influence of drugs. A careful analysis of the manuscripts of Wilkie Collins' The Moonstone, and Sir Walter Scott's The Bride of Lammermoore, two works reputed to have been written under the influence of opium, seem to have been largely written and completed before or after periods of illness requiring the use of opium. Similarly there is evidence from the correspondence of the authors themselves that both Jack Kerouac and William Burroughs preferred to write the bulk of their work without drugs."[87]

People are nourished by experiences, encounters, and reflections that are not necessarily related to their current task or activity. Psychoactive substances can be a way to broaden the human experience, to open the doors of perception, to deepen the palette of emotions, to dive into the unknown to find something new. These altered states of consciousness, these states of mind, these experiences that go from mystical transport to decay, will serve as material, as a support for creation, but often at a distance.

Antoine Perpère, curator of the exhibition "Sous influences. Artists and Psychotropic Drugs"[96] , proposes in the book dedicated to this exhibition to separate the position of artists in relation to these experiences into three categories: Translate, Simulate and Represent.

New sensations, new emotions but also new knowledge; Henri Michaux, great poet, will draw from his experiments with psychotropic substances works such as "Miserable Miracle" or "Knowledge by the chasms" of which we deliver here an extract:

"Drugs bore us with their paradise.

Let them give us some knowledge instead.

We are not a century in paradise.

Any drug changes your support. The support you used to have on your senses, the support your senses used to have on the world, the support you used to have on your general feeling of being. They give way. A vast redistribution of sensibility takes place, which makes everything strange, a complex, continuous redistribution of sensibility. You feel less here, and more there. Where "here"? Where "there"? In dozens of "here", in dozens of "there", that you did not know, that you do not recognize. Obscure zones that were clear. Light areas that were heavy. It is no longer you that you end up with, and reality, the objects themselves, losing their mass and stiffness, cease to offer any serious resistance to the omnipresent transforming mobility.

Abandonments appear, small ones (the drug tickles you with abandonments), big ones too. Some like it. Paradise, that is to say abandonment. You undergo multiple, different invitations to let go... This is what strong drugs have in common and also that it is always the brain that takes the hits, that observes its backstage, its strings, that plays small and big games, and that, afterwards, takes a step back, a singular step back."[97]

V.4. The artist and his environment: a risk factor?

After having approached the couple substances/art with the idea that the substances influence the various stages of the artistic process, we wish to turn over, in a way perhaps a little artificial, our angle of approach. Is the artist, because he creates, because of what it implies, because he is an artist and asserts himself as such, more likely to use substances? To examine this idea let us question the fact that psychoactive substances could less influence the process of creation itself than participate in the "balance" of the artist.

Being an artist can bring a lot of pleasure and even happiness but it is not an easy job. The creation, the relationship with the public, generates sufferings, anguishes, that the artist can be tempted to appease by using drugs and alcohol. The bohemian life, often precarious, is confused with some risk factors of addictions. Finally, artists, like the rest of society, can be influenced by the socio-cultural aspect of myths, such as that of the "cursed artist".

V.4.1. The creative process can generate anxieties

In the previous section, we mentioned very quickly the idea that psychoactive substances could be used to stop the creative process, to relax after a demanding work. We can go further and affirm that creation can be responsible for major psychic tensions, and that drugs can be an attempt at "self-medication" for the suffering and difficulties that are generated.

This is the opinion of Rauch who tells us in the article "the poet syndrome": "Visiting the unknown and stretching the boundaries of reason, creates, for some, the need to use psychotropic substances, to alleviate the stress generated by this kind of activity.[98]

R. Roussillon also insists on the suffering generated by creation: "The release of defenses cannot be envisaged without sufficient security insofar as it is accompanied by an important vulnerability. It is a question "of finding again, at least partly, the affects and internal states charged with displeasure which accompanied the uncreated experience." If it was necessary to the creator to withdraw from the primitive experience it is because it generated "affects often extreme, accompanied by impotence, distress, loneliness." "[99]

Finally D. Knafo expands on this idea, and speaks of the potential difficulties of emotional abandonment and the plunge into the unconscious: "Drug use may represent for artists a way of dealing with a specific anxiety that would be aroused by the creative process itself. The "regressive pull" that occurs during the creative process brings with it great anxiety. The true acceptance of such emotional abandonment means that the artist is under threat of loss of self, loss of reality, loss of control, and possible reactivation of trauma. Coming into contact with unconscious material is not always something pleasant, and may require the artist to confront spiritual danger, to risk feelings of anxiety, terror and rage. Such an encounter can be fraught with primal fears, often felt in terms of life and death. The anxiety generated by the creative process can reach paralyzing levels, and some artists use substances to try to lower it to a level that allows the creative work to continue."[85]

The creative process ultimately leads to a relationship with the public that can be a particular moment of tension. One thinks of course of the stage fright of actors or musicians, but more generally, and without necessarily performing physically in public, the fact of subjecting one's creation to the signature, to the gaze of others, to criticism, can be accompanied by a procession of fears and anguish.

This stage is part of the process and even constitutes, for D. Anzieu, the fifth stage: "Unconscious resistance returns in force with the fifth and final moment of the work of creation: to declare the work finished, to detach it definitively from oneself, to expose it to an audience, to face judgments, criticisms - or worse still, indifference -, to accept for it the risk of having only an ephemeral survival, or this other risk, that it leads from now on a life of its own, different from the one that the creator had hoped to put in it. Many creators keep their manuscripts in a drawer for a long time, unhook their paintings on the day of the opening, forbid the re-publication of their works, the projection of films dating from a period of their existence that they reject, burn their paintings, break their sculptures, demand from their heirs the non-preservation and non-publication, not only of their intimate papers, drafts, sketches, but of works that they consider unfinished."[1]

V.4.2. The living conditions of the artist

The hypothesis here is that artistic professions are most often accompanied by unfavorable socio-economic conditions that may be risk factors for addiction.

The economic conditions of the artists lead P.M. Menger to speak about the "dark picture of the socio-economic curse of the artists". In this article "Rationality and Uncertainty in the Life of an Artist"[100] , we can read that "if the uncertainty of success contributes to the social prestige of the artistic professions and to the very magic of a type of activity that has become the paradigm of free, non-routine, ideally fulfilling work, it also generates considerable disparities in condition between those who succeed and those who are relegated to the lower degrees of the pyramid of fame."

The acceptance of such risks lies in the hope of non-monetary benefits and is related to the fact that "the values respectively attached to social integration through regular, normally paid activity, and to free disposal in the ordinarily painful experience of unemployment, are as if reversed, to celebrate the benefits of that particular species of work, art, ideally fulfilling but socially risky, and to reject the disadvantages of economically safer but more routine and utilitarian occupations."

The particularities of the labor market for artists and their consequences represent an individual fragility of artists linked to a double precariousness. In addition to the precariousness linked to the status of the job, linked to the nature of the work itself but also to the growth in supply (for example, 23,000 musician-performers in 1999 as opposed to 12,000 in 1982), their situation pushes many musicians to accept jobs on the periphery of their profession, "food" jobs, achieving what the author calls a precariousness of "identity"[101] .

Another hypothesis is that the lack of a structured lifestyle designed to maintain stability and minimize change may represent a stressful, psychic cost related to the stigma of being different.[102]

We can see from these few examples that the conditions and rhythms of artists' lives can be associated with precariousness, poverty and stress, which may correspond to certain vulnerability factors common to addictions.

V.4.3. The influence of the myth of the artist under influence

The myth of the artist using psychoactive substances can influence artists. If the "symbolic filiation to a recognized creator" that Anzieu spoke of in our very first chapter is with a person known for his or her use of psychoactive substances, he or she will probably be encouraged to experiment with them in turn. More generally, there is no lack of examples of artists using psychoactive substances and they can constitute a form of model for a young artist.

A substance can also be part of a cultural movement and influence those who are or want to be part of it. The example of heroin with bebop is striking and in an article[90] devoted to this subject one can for example read the testimony of Red Rodney (member of Charlie Parker's quintet): "Heroin was our badge. It was what gave us membership in a single club. And for that membership, we gave up everything else in the world. It ruined most people."

The figure of Charlie Parker comes back in this testimony reported by Stan Getz: "The use of heroin became almost a rite of passage among young jazz musicians (...) and one of the reasons was the example of Charlie Parker. Beyond the myth of Charlie Parker, we can feel in this example the influence of the peer group, the social group to which the creator belongs.

V.5. Common roots

In our endeavor to "unpack" the different and varied relationships between creativity and substance use, we have previously focused on the influences they exert on each other. We assumed that if both were present, then one was generated or simply facilitated by the other. This approach has allowed us to put forward some explanations and insights. The path we are now going to follow is that of deeper phenomena, which would be responsible for both creativity and the use of psychoactive substances.

When we analyze the characteristics of creative people and those with substance use disorders, when we cross-reference the data from the first chapters of this book, we find a number of commonalities. We will first outline these common characteristics. Suffering, trauma, sensitivity can encourage the use of art... or of psychoactive substances. Certain personality traits, mental disorders, are also overrepresented in both types of population.

V.5.1. Suffering, grief and trauma

The idea that deficiencies, suffering, past traumas can be a driving force for creation is quite commonly accepted. It is in general case studies or lists of artists having suffered from the loss of their parents, physical deformity or emotional trauma of all kinds that support these theories. We owe its most direct and violent expression to

Antonin Artaud: "No one has ever written or painted, sculpted, modeled, built, invented, except to get out of hell.

The link between addiction and suffering is very often put forward. Thus, according to the title of M. Valleur and J.C. Matysiak's book, addictions would be a new way of thinking (or of healing) psychological suffering.

An American study[103] tracking adolescents contacted 1,753 people by telephone and studied, in addition to standard demographics, their trauma history, focusing on sexual assault, physical assault, severe physical punishment, witnessing violence, post-traumatic stress disorder, substance use or abuse, and family history of substance use or abuse. The results show that trauma increases the risk of substance use disorders for both men and women. The risk increases even in the absence of Post Traumatic Stress Disorder itself.

In an article entitled "the psychic economy of addiction"[55] , J. McDougall insists on the fact that "addictive solutions" are most often responses to try to get rid of psychic tensions, suffering, guilt, sadness... and that it is almost always "a response to a psychic suffering from the past... a childish attempt to cure oneself. After some clinical vignettes, she concludes by saying: "As no element or object belonging to the real world can repair the lacks in the internal psychic world, the addictive behavior inevitably suffers from a compulsive dimension.

We move away a little from the title of the chapter, but there is here an interesting link to evoke between addictions and art. Addictions can be an attempt to find the lost paradise of childhood, whether by the addictive process itself, or in a more "pharmacological" way, by the effects of certain drugs giving a new freshness, a certain naivety in the look. "The victims of addiction are all engaged in a struggle against the universal dependencies of human beings, including the illusion of rediscovering the lost paradise of childhood, freedom, the absence of any responsibility and the notion of time.[55] Picasso said that he had put all his life to know how to draw like a child, Baudelaire that "the genius, it is the childhood found at will" and beyond beautiful quotations, the relation of the art to the childhood is very rich and complex, and this relation, this attraction towards the childhood can thus be considered as one of the roots common to both phenomena.

V.5.2. The sensitivity

Sensitivity is, according to the dictionary "Trésor de la langue française", the "faculty of deeply feeling impressions, of experiencing feelings, of living an intense affective life".

The sensitivity of the artists is a common place, it is intrinsic to their work. In this same dictionary we find a particular definition of the sensitivity for the artists: "faculty to feel feelings and aptitude to translate them, to express them in an artistic creation" and by metonymy, to speak about the "quality of a work where are manifested and expressed with force the feelings of the artist".

Concerning addictions, the idea is also widespread. For example, we quote Dr. Lowenstein: "the common factor of all the addicted patients who come to see me is, without any hesitation, hypersensitivity. They are emotionally ill"[104] , in the epilogue of the same book we can read "After more than twenty years of clinical practice, the only etiological certainty I have can be summed up in this simple observation: addictions concern above all "hypersensitive" people. Indeed, when I try to remember the thousands of patients that my team and I have met and treated, a common trait emerges: the vast majority of them are people "on edge", in a state of permanent cogitation and rumination". We can see from this excerpt that the sensitivity the author is talking about is not entirely superimposable on the definition of artistic sensitivity, but the two ideas are intertwined and could be a common root.

V.5.3. Personality and psychopathology

We will go into some detail in the first chapters. By comparing the personality traits and the information concerning the psychiatric disorders presented in the beginning of our work, some similarities have emerged. In the analysis of the personality of the two populations, we will note first of all the openness to experiences, the search for novelty, but also the impulsiveness and the taste for transgression.

Under certain conditions, in certain cases, mental disorders could promote creativity. The links between psychotropic substances and psychopathology are very close. Personality disorders or psychiatric pathologies can be the source of both great artistic creativity and substance use.

V.6. Common wings?

"ENJOY"

"You have to be drunk all the time. Everything is there: that is the only question. In order not to feel the horrible burden of Time that breaks your shoulders and bends you towards the Earth, you must get drunk without ceasing.

But of what? Wine, poetry or virtue, as you wish. But get drunk.

And if sometimes, on the steps of a palace, on the green grass of a ditch, in the dreary solitude of your room, you wake up, the intoxication already diminished or gone, ask the wind, the wave, the star, the bird, the clock, everything that flees, everything that groans, everything that rolls, everything that sings, everything that speaks; ask what time it is ; and the wind, the wave, the star, the bird, the clock, will answer you: "It's time to get drunk! To avoid being the martyred slaves of Time, get drunk; get drunk all the time! With wine, poetry or virtue, as you wish." *Charles Baudelaire, short prose poems n°XXXIII*[105]

This poem is remarkable for its poetic qualities, and it also illustrates wonderfully the idea developed in this section. The common roots we have been talking about so far are, to use a term that is popular in the medical field, risk factors. On this ground, the missions, the objectives that individuals assign to art and to psychoactive substances are the same. The other important point is the parallel made in the possible solutions: wine, poetry, virtue...

V.6.1. Fulfilling common existential functions ?

What do a creative process and the consumption of psychoactive substances have in common? From the common ground mentioned above, the parallel is to be found in the goals set: to face emotions, to manage them, to escape suffering, to envisage death and the emptiness of existence, and despite everything to seek pleasure, joy and to build one's life in a positive way. We can identify three axes: controlling the negative, facing questions and moving towards the positive. In this part we will review different common functions that psychotropic substances and artistic creation can try to fulfill.

Managing emotions

The use of psychoactive substances can be seen as a way to manage emotions. According to the one which will be used, the effect could be a decrease of the intensity, an anaesthesia, an exacerbation or a discovery. The artist, for his part, has a singular relationship to emotions which hold an essential place in his work. Thus, Picasso said that "The artist is a receptacle of emotions coming from anywhere, from the sky, from the earth, from a piece of paper, from a passing figure, from a spider's web."

Alleviating suffering

Psychoactive substances and art are consolations of the pain of living. We have spoken in the common roots of the sufferings, the mournings and the past traumas. Art can be an attempt to get out of it. The psychoactive substances can be seen as attempts of self-medication. The destruction or transformation of this negativity can be common goals.

"Facing death

The psychological sufferings mentioned in the previous paragraphs are not always pathological. There is a suffering, a universal drama that concerns all humans: the inexorable passage of time, and then death. His own death, his confrontation and the death of those he loves... It is a very unpleasant prospect and everyone tries to cope with it as best they can.

In this attempt, art and psychotropic drugs have a special place. The use of certain drugs allows for an experience of near death and resurrection. Some people have come close to death through their excessive consumption and claim it. Marc Valleur defines ordalic behaviour as follows: "the fact that a subject engages more or less repeatedly in trials involving a mortal risk: ordeal whose outcome should not be obviously foreseeable and which is distinguished from suicide pure and simple as well as from the simulacrum" and "the ordalic fantasy would be the fact of putting oneself in the hands of the other, to the chance, to the destiny, to the luck, to master it or to be the chosen one, and, by its survival, to show all its right to the life, if not its exceptional character, can be its immortality".

The author describes the characteristics of this type of behaviour, some of which we have already discussed: a subjective relationship to risk or a transgressive aspect. It is on this illusion of mastery of death that we want to insist.

J. Mcdougall also talks about the relationship to death in addiction phenomena: "Finally, the final defiance is to death itself, and this takes two directions: the first proclaims brazenly "nothing touches me, death is for others!"; but when this noisy form of defense collapses and the sensation of internal death can no longer be denied, one discovers a submission before the death drives ("the next shot may be an overdose, but I don't care")."

Art can also be seen as an attempt to thwart the fate of death. It is around the funeral rites, since the Paleolithic, with the Neanderthal man, that it finds one of its first expressions, and thereafter, with the Taj Mahal or the pyramids of Egypt, one of its most sparkling illustrations. If I paint my beloved, her image will never die, if I compose a piece for her, the pianists who will play it in ten generations will revive our love. This attempt may seem vain, but in a more general way it is the artist, the author, who survives through his work in the collective memory of men, it is through what he leaves them that he enters history, that he belongs to the heritage of humanity and becomes eternal.

Filling the void of life

Life that is not yet lived has no real existence. Between the present moment and death there is nothing... for the moment. This future space is probably determined, at least in part, but it is nonetheless uncertain. The man who is, in the present, at the edge of this space and who looks at the void, can be seized by a vertigo which can incite him to develop strategies. One of them is the repetition, the cycle which, predictable, potentially infinite, fills and reassures. One could consider creation under this angle of repetition from work to work, but it is especially a central element of addictions. Artistic creation could be an attempt to fill this space in other ways, by the creation of a real and lasting object for example, but more generally by populating nothingness, by creating or inventing from nothing, it could represent a way to accept the emptiness of our existence.

At the junction between the questions evoked previously and that of pleasure, one could evoke another common function, that of knowledge. "There are artists who, deliberately, are interested in the practice above all, as place of existential, relational, spiritual experiments, or as occasion of social or political action, of technical invention, of metaphysical reflection..."[106] . One can also consider the psychoactive substances as instruments of knowledge, and we refer, for example, to the text of Henri Michaux quoted above.[97]

Achieving pleasure and joy

In contrast to the anguish and suffering on the hedonic spectrum, it is assumed that man seeks to move towards pleasure, joy, happiness, rather than the opposite. Psychoactive substances and artistic creation can be seen as tools, not only to neutralize what one does not want, but to achieve what one wants. The pleasures and joys caused by certain substances are well known, we will not dwell on the subject. The links between creativity and pleasure are deep and it will be interesting to watch four ten-minute videos entitled: "Pleasure in artistic creation" (on a well-known video search engine). They include nine interviews with Quebec artists and illustrate strong, multiple and complex links. Finally, if these links with pleasure exist, the path is strewn with pitfalls: not all artists are fulfilled, and some substance users, caught in a spiral of addiction, have, in the long term, the opposite effect to the one sought.

To conclude, by highlighting that there are two practices that respond to the same functions, we want to emphasize that each of them can be a contribution, and not necessarily always fulfill all these functions. In view of the nature of the problems raised, it seems sensible to multiply the strategies. This is precisely one of the problems with addictions: the reduction to a single solution. Faced with a problem (anxiety, sadness, boredom, lack of pleasure, sensations...), the motivation to choose the "addictive solution" will be more and more important.

V.6.2. Psychoanalysis: transformation of narcissism

By confronting the psychoanalytical approaches of creation and addictions, we have noted the recurrence of the idea of narcissism. Narcissism is, by reference to the myth of Narcissus, the love of one's own image. In psychoanalytical terms, it is the investment of libido on the subject himself.

The failing narcissistic foundations and their origins were somewhat detailed in the chapter on addictions. If certain psychoactive substances are used in these circumstances, it is because they contribute, at least for a time, to recovering this "original narcissistic dimension" of the self, by raising the affective tone, by improving self-esteem and by temporarily ensuring sufficient "inner security".

But we will especially take advantage of this chapter to bring elements of reflections on the links which can exist between creativity, art and narcissism.

Raskin[107] uses the second part of the Barron Symbolic Equivalent test as well as self-declarations to evaluate the creativity of 71 students and divide them into 4 groups. He then uses a narcissistic personality test, the Narcissic Personality Inventory. The results show a weak but significant relationship, showing in particular a higher "narcissistic score" in people who are more creative and declare themselves to be more creative than those who are less creative and declare themselves not to be.

Kohut argues that "if artists and scientists can crave acclaim, if they can be narcissistically vulnerable individuals, if their ambition can be to encourage themselves through appropriate communication about their work, creativity itself deserves to be considered among the transformations of narcissism"[108] . It should be noted that in the same article he counts as other transformations of narcissism empathy, wisdom or humor.

The transformation of narcissism is for him to be sought in the relation of the artist with his creation. The narcissistic energy is transformed into "idealizing libido", that is to say the elaboration of this point in the development that goes from narcissism to object love, this point where the object is invested with the narcissistic libido, thus incorporating it into the self. For creative people, their work is a transitional object, invested with a narcissistic transitional libido. Creative people have, according to Kohut, a narcissistic experience of the world (an extended self encompassing the world). "Creative artists and scientists may be attached to their work in the manner of an addiction, they try to control it and shape it with forces and goals that belong to a narcissistic experience of the world."[108]

V.6.3. Neurobiological aspects: the example of anti-parkinsonian treatments

In the same way as for psychoanalysis, we will choose to develop only one track relating to the comparison of creativity and addictions on the neurobiological level. This is the role of dopamine and the example given to us in this respect by the results of the treatment of Parkinsonian patients.

Treatment of patients with Parkinson's disease with dopamine agonists or L-Dopa can cause impulse control disorders (pathological gambling, hypersexuality, punding, compulsive eating and shopping...) sometimes grouped under the term Dopamine Dysregulation Syndrome. These disorders have an obvious relationship with addictions and for some of them they can be related to addictions without psychoactive substances.

A 2010 study of 3090 patients[109] shows an association between impulse control disorders of all types and antiparkinsonian treatment. Although an association was shown for L-Dopa use, agonist use had a greater risk and the combination of L-Dopa with an agonist still greatly increased the risk. An Australian review from 2010[110] gathers 19 studies and finds a causal link between antiparkinsonian treatment (in particular dopaminergic agonist) and impulse control disorders. Between 4 and 13.6% would develop such disorders, which corresponds to a factor of 6 compared to the general population. The level of evidence is higher for pathological gambling.

What is the relationship between anti-parkinsonian treatments and creativity? We have seen in the section on creativity that taking L-Dopa and Benserazide, a peripheral dopadecarboxylase inhibitor, led to an increase in the signal-to-noise ratio and a decrease in the remoteness of associations in the context of a lexical decision test. However, evidence from clinical practice with Parkinson's patients seems to contradict this conclusion and many articles report increased creativity under treatment.[111-114]

What are the mechanisms of this increase? Various hypotheses have been put forward: psychodynamic, with a sublimation process linked to the announcement of the disease; behavioural disinhibition which may or may not be linked to the treatment (for example, disruption of inhibition latency[112]); pre-morbid personality revealed by the restoration of a dopaminergic balance; creativity linked to serotonergic hyperstimulation[111] The very nature of the treatment and the chronology seem to indicate an effect of dopaminergic agonists.

A study compared 36 Parkinson's patients, half of whom were considered to have increased creative activities under treatment (more than two hours per day after introduction of the treatment), with 36 "control" patients.[113] Creativity was studied by the Torrance test, impulsivity by the Barratt Impulsiveness Scale and the Minnesota Impulsive Disorders Interview. The results were in the direction of an increase in motivation to create (motivation towards the hedonic properties of creation) with a normalized creativity (joining that of the population

control). This increase in artistic activities was not related to an increase in impulsivity or impulse control disorders.

6. Discussion

There comes a point when you have to stop untangling the balls and try to weave something together. We spent the first parts of this book clarifying our ideas about the protagonists, then trying to get a clearer and more orderly idea of their relationships. Now we need to think about their implications for medicine and care. In this discussion we will present reflections from the previous chapters and present existing work on the subject.

VI.1 Some ideas for reflection

We create our own life

The fact that life is a work is an old idea. Even if his thought is more complex and to be put in a particular context, we can retain the image of Plotinus: "never stop sculpting your own statue". Closer to us, Michel Foucault said, in a conference pronounced in Berkley: "What astonishes me, it is the fact that in our society the art became something which is in connection only with the objects and not with the individuals or with the life (...). But couldn't the life of every individual be a work of art? Why is a lamp or a house an art object and not our life?

There are constraints influencing this creation

We lead our life, we try to fill it, to create it, to build it in the best way possible. However, life is not a blank page, our freedom is not complete.

We have seen in the previous chapter that artistic creation and the use of psychoactive substances can be considered as two strategies to control the negative, the suffering, to face questions, fears, anxieties and to go towards the positive, towards pleasure. These are universal objectives and in the perspective of building one's existence, these objectives can be seen as natural guidelines. Of course, there are obstacles to reach these goals, they are subject to calculations, the means used can conflict with other constructions, moral or social, and all these constraints solicit our creativity.

Alongside these underlying objectives, there are other constraints. We have our own characteristics, our personality, our skills, our body, but also our past, our wounds, our sufferings.

Secondly, our life has a reality in a material environment that never ceases to influence us: the climate, the light, the nature...

Finally, in this environment, there are other individuals who are also creating their lives and with whom we interact. There is our family and more generally the various societies which form the Men and in which we evolve.

Rather than a blank page, we see that the creation of our life takes place in the midst of a proliferation of influences, relationships, and constraints, on which we are dependent. J. Mc Dougall tells us that "dependence is an intrinsic part of the human condition. We begin with a dependency on the mother-breast universe, continue to be caught up in a series of dependencies, even if we are not always aware of it, in that human nature seeks to live in conformity with the socio-cultural standards in which it is immersed. We are therefore all dependent on and subject to a series of collective ideals that are the basis of any social contract. We have not asked for anything because it has always existed, but we are obliged to submit to this dependence. We are also obliged to accept the ravages of the time, as, besides, to be dependent on the language that exercises on our psychosexual construction and our psychological structure an indelible mark. In short, the dependence is our destiny, as well as the incessant and inhuman fight that we lead against it to try to escape from it. "[55]

The problem of addictions

In the context of medicine, the case that interests us in particular and that we will develop is that of patients suffering from addiction problems. One of the problems they encounter is the increasingly important place that these practices take in their lives, until their entire existence revolves around them.

If one puts oneself in the perspective of the creation of one's existence, one sees that at a given moment, the person has built himself through a set of practices, that he has attributed to them certain roles, certain functions, but that they have ended up being harmful to him. It is then necessary to try to build oneself in another way or even to rebuild oneself and the artistic creation can have a role to play for this purpose.

The substitution

The most obvious path is that of substitution. We can imagine that where substances have taken all the place, where they answer all the problems, artistic creation can offer an alternative solution. It is not a question of making artistic practices THE new solution but rather of integrating them as one of the possible "substitute" solutions.

A good way to build yourself is to build something.

We can also imagine that these artistic practices will help patients to rebuild their lives as they wish, with or without art. Beyond being a substitute, they would allow to have a new look on all these constraints and to acquire skills to be able to consider them differently, with or without art. In this case we would no longer be in a form of translation, of construction of oneself through different things, but rather in a multiplication of constructions: one builds a work, one finishes it, one builds another one, one improves one's capacities of creation, expression, resolution of problems... We acquire skills, we develop ideas, we improve faculties that are useful in the construction of our life.

Relationship to the world, relationship to others, relationship to oneself

These skills concern several aspects of our lives. First of all, the relationship with the world. We have seen that sensitivity is an important characteristic of patients suffering from addictions. This can be modified by substances and we can imagine that artistic practices allow to cultivate, to analyze, to work on emotions, where sensations had imposed themselves.

Then the relationship with others is fundamental. Communication and expression difficulties are a major problem that can be considered as a cause and a consequence of addiction problems. Art can allow people to express themselves, we speak of artistic expression, a work exists through the eyes of the spectator. The creation is sometimes done in group. We can therefore imagine a positive action of an artistic expression work on this aspect of the problem.

Finally, artistic creation can, on several levels, change one's relationship to oneself. The relationship we have with others and with the world around us depends on us, but it is more precisely the image, the esteem, that we have of ourselves, which can be improved through an artistic practice. This one also makes it possible to question oneself in depth, consciously or not (for example in the research of material of creation), and by there to know oneself better and finally to modify one's own relationship to oneself, by structuring oneself by the interior without contribution of external object.

Suffering and pleasure

In addiction problems, the pleasure that a behavior provoked at the beginning of its history gradually fades away, suffering takes over and we witness a spiral of distress. As we explained in the previous chapter, art can help to combat and transform suffering, to "get out of hell". On the other hand, the provoked pleasure can be intense and prolonged, but it is not systematic nor necessarily where we expect it.

These are a few angles of approach, a few paths that suggest that through artistic practices, one can contribute to filling one's life, to creating it, to building it differently, in a way that is both more structured and more diverse. These practices also seem particularly adapted to certain problems encountered in addictions.

Framing

As we have already mentioned, an artist puts himself in danger when he searches deep inside himself, when he excites and exacerbates his sensibility, when he delivers his productions to the critics and the public. It therefore seems judicious to evaluate the indications and to frame these practices if we want to be effective and if we want to avoid aggravating the situation.

Prevention

We had in mind, when talking about addiction problems, the case of addicted people, suffering from these problems and trying to get out of them, but we could very well consider that artistic practices are tools of prevention. Indeed, the creation of one's own existence concerns each of us, and the different positive aspects we have talked about apply to everyone and could contribute to prevent the installation of addictive disorders.

The relationship between artistic creation and therapy is very old, and recent studies continue to shed light on their links, even if in the field of addictions the literature is not abundant. The practical application of artistic practices in a therapeutic framework exists within the framework of art-mediated therapies. We will therefore devote the remainder of this discussion to confronting the ideas outlined so far with the articles found in our research.

VI.2 General information on art therapy

Even before pointing out the difficulties of a definition, it is important to note the difficulty of agreeing on the term art therapy. There is indeed a plethora of more or less similar semantic variations designating more or less similar practices. Art and/or therapy, psychotherapies mediated to/with artistic/expressive/creative mediations are used in French[115] , but there is also a profusion of pseudo-synonyms in other languages[116] . The term art therapy is vague but is the most frequently used.

VI.2.1. History

A brief historical overview will allow us to better understand what art-mediated therapies are today. There have been links between art and therapy at least since antiquity. From the XIXème century onwards, the links between art and psychiatry became more obvious. J.P Klein proposes four sources of "art therapy"[117] . Firstly, art was seen as a means of diversion (which he likens to the work of the insane advocated by Pinel and then to the current of "occupational" therapies). It has also been considered as a means of expression, of releasing tensions, of catharsis.

Secondly, art seen as decoding. He traces this source back to Charcot with "Les démoniaques dans l'art". Freud followed this line with "A childhood memory of

Leonardo da Vinci". Later, we can quote Robert Volmat, who founded the Society of Psychopathology of Expression. Art has here a semiological value.

Thirdly, sometimes blending with the previous one, a current insists more on the aesthetic value of the artistic productions of people suffering from mental disorders. Hans Prinzhorn and his collection are one of the emblems, later Dubuffet and the art brut give another illustration.

The fourth and last trend is that of child psychiatry, which has used drawings since the beginning, sometimes for therapeutic purposes.

More simply, other authors identify two traditions, two approaches that continue to this day.[115,116,118] One advocates a cathartic practice, with an accompaniment of creation. This current is represented by Adrian Hill and Edith Kramer and defends a practice of "art as therapy". The other current can be represented by Margaret Naumburg, who insists more on the interpretative recovery, and conceives rather a practice of "art in therapy". The two currents are not incompatible in practice.[115]

VI.2.2. Definition

The French federation of art therapists has the simplest definition: "Art therapy is a care practice based on the therapeutic use of the process of artistic creation." The Larousse definition of art therapy is more precise: "an approach

of accompanying a person or a group, centered on the expression of oneself, one's thoughts, emotions and conflicts in an artistic creation process."

If we look across the Channel we find the definition of the British Association of Art Therapists (BAAT), which provides further elements: it is a psychotherapy that uses art as the primary means of communication; patients do not need to have any previous skills or experience in the arts; the therapist's main goal is neither an aesthetic nor a diagnostic assessment; the goal is for the patient to grow personally, in a supportive and safe environment, through the use of artistic materials.

Before defining art-mediated therapy, J.P. Klein points out the limits of the different currents from which it originates in order to say what it is not.[117]

- It is not the psychotherapy with artistic support that continues to be in /I/ but with other languages than the verbal language: self-portrait, self-narrative, theatrical representation of its own fear, modulation of its complaint in song, all then verbalized and analyzed

- It is not a diagnostic or semiological test in psychiatric or psychoanalytical terms

- It is not a simple sensitization to the art which consists in a discovery of the matter which would not be an indirect projective work on oneself incited by triggers of personal implication

- It is not a leisure and entertainment activity.

For him, creation is seen as a process of transformation. He defines art therapy as follows: "Therapeutic accompaniment of people placed in a position of creation so that their journey from work to work becomes a process of transformation of themselves. He gives us a shorter version: "Therapeutic accompaniment of people, generally in difficulty, through the production of artistic works".

VI.3 Literature review

Searches were conducted on various databases: pubmed, APA psycARTICLES, Google scholar, Taylor and Francis, ScienceDirect. The keywords used were: art therapy, mediation therapy, addiction; and in English: art therapy, substance use /related disorder, addiction.

We encountered several difficulties: in particular, the profusion of articles, many of which were not relevant: if we search for the words "art therapy" and "substance related disorder", we mainly find articles concerning the treatment of HIV by antiretroviral treatment, which is known as ART in English. We also found many articles containing the term "State of Art". Where possible, we used filters or keywords (e.g. Mesh). We then tried to identify the most relevant articles by reading the abstracts, and we were able to discover other articles, one after another and from bibliography to bibliography. We must specify from the outset, that we were not able to have access to the full text of all the articles, and we will therefore not mention them.

The results in French language were quite few and those in English language represented the main part of our sources. The articles concerning the analysis of the works of people suffering from addictions were discarded, in order to remain focused on the treatment. In total, we were able to analyze more than thirty articles and some chapters of several books. We found three reviews of the literature proper, one of which was devoted exclusively to music, but several articles began with a section devoted to existing work.

We have identified several areas of focus in analyzing these articles; these are to answer certain questions. First, what are the specific problems of patients with addiction problems and what are the benefits of art therapy? Secondly, how do mediated therapies fit into a more holistic approach? Third, what are the practical modalities? Fourth, what are the results and research perspectives?

VI.3.1. What impacts? Which openings?

We have identified some major recurring themes. We will mention them and illustrate them with a few examples while trying to avoid being redundant.

V I.3.1.1. The implication

To begin with, it should be noted that art is seen as a way to connect with patients. For example, we can read that "art therapy makes it possible to reach patients through art that it is not always possible to reach otherwise."[119] Even more than a contact, art can facilitate the involvement of the patient: "The important thing is the impulse, the involvement of the patient, the vital impetus instilled by the artistic creation."[120]

V I.3.1.2. Expression, communication, the central place of emotions

The first review of the literature, dating from 1983, is based on 20 articles[121.]. It offers a good overview of the themes that will be developed. The emphasis is on the characteristics of people suffering from addictions, which make an intervention by art-mediated therapies particularly favourable. These characteristics are: avoidance of feelings; communication difficulties, which are of two types: defensive use of words and difficulties in conveying feelings verbally; and the need for a non-threatening means of expression. "Self-expression through artistic mediation provides a way around communication and expression difficulties."

"More distanced [by mediation], communication can be perceived as less dangerous and intrusive. A therapeutic alliance is then easier to establish."[122] The safe, non-threatening framework of art, as compared to speech, is regularly emphasized, not only for expressing emotions, but also for communicating in a general way.

The central role of emotions and their expression is found in many articles. Thus, mediated therapies can help "treat alexithymia, the inability to translate bodily tensions into images, to represent feelings"[123] . "Art therapy seems a unique way in the field [of addiction] to explore and express emotions that are felt to be overwhelming."[124] " [Patients] are able to express thoughts and feelings in images that they might otherwise never have discovered or revealed."[125] ; "Art is particularly helpful because of its non-verbal nature. Because developmental frustrations were experienced before verbalization, many narcissistic patients are unable to verbalize their feelings. [...] Artistic expression represents a safe step toward eventual verbal discharge."[126]

We have seen that certain factors of addictions are located in the past of individuals, and if certain authors refuse a return on possible traumas or frustrations, others on the other hand allow it. Thus, in the previous paragraph, we speak of "exploring", "discovering or revealing". In a more general way: "Art therapy can be used as an instrument of self-knowledge. And the more one knows about oneself, the better equipped one is to change negative behavior patterns."[119]

V   I.3.1.3. The defenses

The problem of defenses is central, even if, as we will come back to, the way to approach it varies. Depending on the authors and the schools of thought, art therapy will allow us to break them down, to "destroy the ramparts of defense", to bypass them or to strengthen them. to circumvent them or to fortify them.[127] Denial is often targeted in the articles, and in an underlying way shame, guilt and loss.[128] For Lynn Johnson, shame is the name of the disease and art is a way to transform it.[129] Alongside denial, other defenses such as minimization, accusation, passivity-aggressivity and projection are also mentioned.[130,131]

V   I.3.1.4. The feeling of control

Art could help the patient regain control over his or her feelings, first by developing artistic skills, and second by creating and manipulating symbols.[121] "The patient can create and master experiences, symbols, and translate them into real life."[132] Art therapy can restore a sense of mastery, pleasure (enjoyment), and physical engagement.[121]

V   I.3.1.5. Self-esteem

Self-esteem is also a theme that recurs in almost every article. For Moore, again in the first review, self-expression and mastery improve self-esteem.[121] In 2007, in the short review that begins his article, Dickinson[133] points out that many authors encourage the improvement of self-esteem through skill development and artistic creativity. Another article states that self-esteem can be improved through dance, accepting limitations and recognizing strengths.[134] Elsewhere, improved self-esteem is presented as an important outcome of group art therapy work, with patients recognizing their displayed work and showing it with pride to their peers.[125]

Some articles emphasize that artistic productions have the advantage of being tangible supports[119] , material, allowing a discussion around a real object, also allowing a documentation of the evolution of the patient, both for him/herself, and for the whole therapeutic team.[135]

To summarize, after having succeeded in approaching the patient and involving him/her, mediation therapies tackle different problems in different ways: firstly recognition, mastery and above all, communication, expression of emotions; secondly defenses; thirdly self-esteem and their component of shame and guilt. The creation would thus allow in turn the knowledge, the expression, the valuation of oneself. These different axes are a way to simplify, to clarify, they can overlap, they can intersect.

VI.3.2. An integration to different theoretical models

Addiction care is complex and multidisciplinary. It can call upon several specialities, several theories, several different techniques, concomitant or sequential. It generally takes place over a fairly long period of time. Not ignoring these data, the articles most often try to present the therapies by artistic mediations, as being part of a larger program, as being able to integrate and have a utility in a larger framework.

VI.3.2.1. The 12 steps

There is a tension that is well explained in the introduction to the special issue of " the Arts in Psychotherapy "[123] on addictions in 1990, a tension between mediated therapies, which have a tradition rooted in psychoanalysis, and a treatment of addictions that is far from it (at least in the United States at that time).

D. Johnson then writes that "art and creative therapies should certainly focus strongly on the Alcoholics Anonymous model and relapse prevention, rather than on a psychodynamic model." He adds a little later that the fundamental question is what art-mediated therapies can contribute to the twelve-step process of AA. His answer is that they can help on several levels. Step one: shame processing; step two: imagining a higher power; step three: taking a thorough moral inventory; step four: bearing witness to others. The improvements in the sense of control, of mastery, mentioned above, can be integrated with cognitive-behavioral therapies, according to him. In addition to the articles in this special issue, the majority of the articles take up this idea of integrating with the twelve steps.

VI.3.2.2. Psychodynamics

The other major tradition, the oldest, is the psychoanalytic tradition. In a 1992 review[124] , Waller and Mahonny note that half of the articles studied use psychoanalytic concepts, but that no one, except Albert-Puelo, delves into the notion of transference. She is also the only one to use the free interview, and the only one to question the interest or not of a structured interview. In this review, the authors point out that in the articles analysed, there are untimely and unjustified changes of method (other than a subjective feeling of failure) and a cruel lack of theoretical references. The most important criticism concerns a "misuse and abuse of the therapeutic relationship" and an almost complete absence of the question of counter-transference.

The psychodynamic notions used in art therapy are rooted in a tradition going back to the pioneers of this discipline. Thus, in his 1981 article[132] , Kaufman recapitulates the history of art therapy to point out the benefits to be expected. Firstly, a mode of introspection and analysis: citing the work of M. Naumburg, she maintains that the artistic productions of patients can play the role of dreams in psychoanalysis. Secondly, and this time relying on E. Kramer: art can be therapeutic in itself. It allows a safe exit for material from the primary process.

Nancy Albert-Puelo, as we have already mentioned, is often quoted as a reference when it comes to art therapy in addiction. What does she tell us in substance?[126] For her, "drug abuse can be seen as an inadequate way to deal with feelings, through withdrawal into euphoric states"; "repeated self-attacks [with drugs] are seen as narcissistic defenses, since narcissistic withdrawal into euphoria allows one to defend against anger and other feelings". She continues: "this way of defending against feelings by blocking them has its roots in early childhood development," in a particularly frustrating environment during the first six months of life. She draws a parallel between drug use and the fact that a small child falls asleep when trying to tolerate extreme frustration. Both are about internalizing aggression or other hostile feelings.

So how do we deal with this kind of problem? After citing the limitations of Freudian ideas in treating narcissistic subjects, she refers to Spotnitz, and writes that "when working with such patients, a narcissistic transference must be encouraged, that is, a transference in which the patient sees the therapist as similar to himself." The goal at this point is "to strengthen the patient's ego by redirecting his or her self-attacks externally through transference," words are welcome, they are not destructive, emotions and feelings can be expressed in a safe setting, without risk of loss. Resistance should be encouraged, as it is useful in life outside of therapy, and once it is no longer needed, it will disappear on its own. Eventually childhood traumas can be re-experienced in treatment, corrections and education can be made, and the energy released can be used more constructively. She concludes by saying that the key is to resolve the barriers to the expression of internalized aggression.

In a much more recent article, Dickinson[133] offers an example of reconciling the two views: psychodynamic and 12-step, within a multidisciplinary approach.

VI.3.2.3. Brief therapy and motivational approaches

In the 2000s, new approaches have emerged. H. Matto shows in an article the compatibility of art-mediated therapies with solution-focused brief therapies.[135] In another article she insists on the behavioral aspect, in particular to manage the periods of "cravings" and to control the triggers. She then highlights the fact that artistic mediations allow the mobilization of the Situationnal Access Memory in addition to the verbal access memory, an interesting contribution in the cognitive-behavioral framework.[136]

But it is especially the trans-theoretical model of change and motivational interviewing that represents a notable change. In a very interesting article, "moving toward gray", Horay develops the links between art therapy, the stages of change model and motivational interviewing, and puts them in perspective with the two main currents we have been talking about. It is clear that the literature linking art to the 12 steps has little to do with motivational interviewing, because the artistic process it describes remains focused on destroying resistance, encouraging helplessness within the addicted individual, and creating a decidedly positive image of recovery. In contrast, art therapy, which is rooted in a psychodynamic understanding of addiction, aims to reinforce psychological defense mechanisms, promote the patient's strengths, and encourage the emergence of ambivalent feelings and thoughts about recovery.

These latter goals are shared by motivational counselors working in the stages of change." He adds, "Art therapy seems particularly well suited to fill the gap between the cognitive-behavioral issues of motivational interviewing and the traditionally psychodynamic focus on the narcissistic clinic." In a 2009 article Holt[131] quotes this last sentence of Horay's in agreement with it, but differs from him when it comes to the incompatibility of motivational interviewing with the 12 steps, she insists that AA promotes self-evaluation. The article goes on to discuss the value of art therapy in the first stages of the cycle, precontemplative and contemplative.

Finally, in practice, are mediation therapies used? An article by Aletratis[137] is devoted to this. A clear separation is made between Art (AT) and Music (MT). The data is obtained by interviewing the staff of 307 randomly selected American addiction treatment facilities. 37.8% of the programs offered AT, 14.7% MT and 11.7% both. For TA, there was a positive and significant association with facilities using the 12 steps and also an association, but less strong, with motivational therapies. There was no association with "medical assistance" or contingency management therapies. Facility size was positively correlated with TA and being Medicaid funded was negatively correlated.

In conclusion of this section, we see that elements of psychodynamics, more or less anchored in a theoretical model, run through the history of the application of art-mediated therapies in addiction from the beginning. Mediated therapies have been seen as allies in the use and application of the 12-step model of Alcoholics Anonymous, but this almost exclusive role has been challenged by the emergence of motivational interviewing therapies, based on the trans-theoretical model of change and other behavioral therapies.

VI.3.3. The practice

As a preamble, it must be emphasized that the role of the well-trained therapist is central if we want to bring a therapeutic effect that goes beyond the occupation.[120,138]

What happens in practice? What are the parameters used? What are the instructions given? In Moore's review[121] , a great heterogeneity in methods was observed in the first decades. From this point of view, things have changed little and diversity still seems to be the rule.

V   I.3.3.1 Group or individual?

From the beginning, the two visions coexist. Even today: Dickinson[133] uses groups and insists that groups allow for the study and work on interpersonal relationships and that the cohesion and camaraderie emerging from groups can be therapeutic in itself. Horay[127] , influenced by motivational interviewing, uses individual sessions. Some therapists use both.

V   I.3.3.2. Which mediation is used?

There are mostly visual arts, using paint, pencils, pastels, ink..., some props: plastic masks, ribbons, clay modeling. There are a few articles using dance[139-141] , movement, several others using music (see Mays[142] for a specific review on music) - and it should be noted that music is regularly mentioned as an adjunct to visual creation. Two articles[130,143] mention theater, and one the use of puppets. Several types of mediation are often used for the same patients.

The choice of technique is important, it must "hook" the narcotic addiction.[120] Kaufmann tells us that the media are more or less structuring and must be adapted to the type of patient: for her, fragmented patients, with blurred boundaries, would benefit from structuring techniques such as pencils, whereas a rigid, obsessive patient would benefit from a less structured technique such as painting or clay modeling (unless, for example, one wishes to reinforce defenses that one considers useful).[132] Dance directly involves the body, its perception, and the perception of the other's body, and seems to bring to light more resistance than with other media.

Dubois offers a clearer view. She insists on a preliminary evaluation of the patient to know if a mediation is indicated and to choose the adequate mediation. She takes into account the patient's tastes, his level of learning in this or that practice, the nature of his psychic defenses, the impact of his symptoms in his relational life, the awareness of his disorders and the degree of difficulty in communicating.[122]

V I.3.3.3. Instructions? What instructions?

The problem of guidelines, of instructions, is of course linked to the general vision that therapists have of the role of art in their practice. We can schematically group them into two categories. First of all, free expression, often with a psychodynamic tinge; sometimes some instructions are introduced and adapted to the patient. The question of interpretation then arises. All the articles mention a verbalization phase, some recommend caution, only one article talks about it in detail. A second group uses specific instructions to illustrate, reinforce and improve the effectiveness of different strategies: twelve steps, stages of change, behavioural techniques. We will see that in practice there is some overlap. We will now look at the different guidelines in a more concrete way, with an inevitable air of catalog.

Albert-Puelo gives us several precise technical indications. The sessions are individual. Interpretations can only take place once the transition from narcissistic transference to object transference has taken place. Interactions should be limited, so as not to over-stimulate or deprive and to avoid counter-transference. She suggests exploring all contacts made by the patient; channeling all actions into words or graphic expression; favoring object-oriented questions over ego-oriented ones; encouraging, working with and welcoming resistance. The parameters: the patient is alone in front of an easel on which a lamp illuminates the white page, like a screen ready to receive projections, the analyst is seated three-quarter behind him.[126]

For Forrest, one cardinal rule: be sober or at least relatively so. For the rest: free painting and group discussions about the works, sometimes using clay, or individual sessions with instructions adapted to the patient: painting his weekend, painting himself on the way to the hospital... always mixed with interviews. For Harms, the basic principle is individual therapy, no instructions are given, often the productions are made outside, brought and discussed in consultation. For him, the support can be done by suggesting a change of technique, or even of field, by showing works in progress or completed, by organizing visits, to the museum, to the show...[120] At Dickinson, the sessions are very free and end with a group discussion about the productions. For Kaufmann[132] , the instructions are more or less structuring and must be adapted to the patient. In the workshops developed by Virshup[125] , the patients dip a string in ink and then slide it over paper, thus creating a surface full of lines of dots, tasks, support for a graphic work using pastels. The productions are titled, a short story accompanies them and they are shared in public.

In Potocek's article[134] we find graphic creations with musical accompaniment, staging, work on "movement" (circle of trust where everyone supports each other, exercise consisting in throwing cushions with different intensities). The objective is to put into practice and reinforce some of the 12 steps. In Feen-Calligan's 1995 groups[144] , sessions began by trying to get patients to feel powerless using various methods, such as drawing with eyes closed with one's non-dominant hand, or drawing in pairs without speaking. Advice on the technical use of the equipment was given, and patients were left free to create or not. Easy access to the tools was provided. Classical music was sometimes played, but the author's preference was for

silence.

In a more recent article by the same author[145] and which takes place during the initial phase of detoxification, specific instructions were given. For example, "draw occasions when you are powerless over alcohol". "Identify and represent triggers for relapse", then pass the paper to a neighbor who will imagine "a solution" to the trigger, and so on until a whole series of possible strategies is obtained. Represent the barriers to recovery with quilting tape, paint a recovery life on top of it, and then remove the tape, illustrating that the composition of a recovery life must take into account the barriers. Specific instructions could be given to explore feelings, such as associating a color with a feeling that precipitated a relapse, drawing a situation where it appears, and writing a short text explaining the importance of exploring that kind of feeling. Shell painting was also done, illustrating the patient's inner and outer worlds and forces. Similar "exercises" were used to represent a healthy life.

Holt presents some guidelines, most often used in groups but also in individuals. "Draw the crisis or incident that brought you into treatment," which is similar to Cox and Price's instruction to "draw an incident that occurred while you were drinking/drug taking"[128] . Another instruction could be: "Draw a bridge and represent where you were, where you are and where you want to go, in relation to your recovery". One exercise, found in Horay[127] , is the "cost-benefit collage," where the patient is asked to represent the positives and negatives of both use and abstinence, an idea taken directly from the principles of motivational interviewing. This article by Holt presents two other possibilities: the portraits in one year, i.e. the portrait with continued use and the portrait without use, and the representation of "the barriers you see to making the changes necessary for recovery".

In addition to the collage presented earlier, Horay suggests beginning each session (individual in this case), by drawing a recently experienced feeling. Another project with the patient presented was that of fictitious thank you cards, which his children could send him.

Matto proposes a very detailed protocol. Some of the instructions have already been mentioned: "draw incidents" or "path to recovery". Add to this: "Draw your addiction", What would it look like if it were an animal? Or if it were three-dimensional? Draw a picture that shows the contrast between what the addiction promises and what it is, between imagination and reality. The detail is mainly carried in the questions that guide the verbal analysis of the productions, they are grouped in four parts: "critical engagement": formal analysis of the production; "initial reactions": subjective analysis of the work; "relational attributes": analysis of the relationships, especially of the patient with the creative process; "building an opportunity for change": part focused on possible solutions.[135]

In another article[136] , Matto gives other possibilities, such as developing the incident drawing in three parts: "before", "during" and "after", in order to break down and highlight the process. Another possibility is a variation of the cost-benefit collage, but with less emphasis on highlighting ambivalence: the representation of the benefits of abstinence and the disadvantages of use. Finally, the use of various materials, magazines, colors, words... to make life-size bodies, one with, the other without substance use, emphasizing emotions and how they act.

In an article on the use of music in patients with a dual diagnosis, Ross[146] gives three possibilities. First, a session that begins with relaxation, then listening to music for twenty minutes, then free graphic expression for another twenty minutes and sharing around these productions for another twenty minutes. Secondly, during a workshop, the patients meet to play percussions. Several phases follow one another, orchestration by the therapist, collective improvisation, playing in small groups, all interspersed with analysis and explanations. Thirdly, a group improvisation with both percussion and melodic instruments. A brief explanation of the use of the instruments is given and the session ends with a verbal analysis.

In terms of theater, Moffet[130] uses film analysis and then play performance, in particular a 20-minute play entitled "Nobody Cares". It highlights and works on defenses.

The whole thing is filmed, which makes it possible to multiply the possibilities of staging and to have a tangible support.

Finally the dance. In Miliken's article[139] the sessions start with a discussion setting limits, rules, explaining the process and purpose of the exercises. After the warm-up, exercises are proposed. Slow movements, focusing on the beginning and the end of the movements, working on the rhythm, are used to work on control. Group exercises, circle exercises, trust exercises are also used. Common exercises can be found in Fisher's article[141] , group dance, confidence exercises, mirror imitation. For Reiland[140] the initial objective is to create a therapeutic link through techniques such as mirroring, then to encourage a process of separation, individuation, to increase the vocabulary of available movements, to gain mastery and control over one's own body, to have a more precise idea of one's body and its boundaries.

VI.3.4. Results and perspectives

We will go rather quickly in this part concerning the results, for the simple reason that the vast majority of the articles analysed say in substance: "it works well, our experiences are good, we should continue in this way, mediation therapies have their place in the treatment of addictions". A subjective positive feeling is encouraging, but we have almost only case analyses and very few attempts to measure a change. It is true that many authors insist on a progressive transformation from work to work. The process is complex, non-linear, sometimes long, and the results cannot be measured in a simple way. Under these conditions, three studies should be noted that are distinguished by their method.

The first is Reiland's, and concerns dance-mediated therapy. The criterion of field dependence or independence (referring to Witkin's work), is studied in four patients, using the ABC (Articulation of the Body Concept) scale to evaluate drawings of human faces by the patients. These drawings were made before and after the first, third and sixth sessions. The results were in the direction of a shift towards field independence (i.e., a more articulated vision, less global, dissociating more easily an element from its context), in the three persons having initially a high field dependence. The results on such a sample are of course not significant, but on the one hand they are interesting and on the other hand the method is also interesting.

The second study is that of Ross[146] , dating from 2008, and concerns music. 80 patients with co-occurring psychiatric disorders were divided into three groups: music and graphic expression, percussion and improvisation. We have previously described these modalities in detail. A series of tests assessed general status, psychiatric symptoms, motivation to change and adherence to treatment, allowing monitoring of patients' progress. Attendance at sessions and patients' attitudes towards music were also assessed.

therapy and towards the therapist were evaluated.

The first result was that no variable at baseline predicted the outcome of the music therapy tests. Another finding was the significant relationship between improvement in overall clinical impression (as measured by the CGI severity scale) and increased music appreciation. Attendance at music therapy sessions was associated with increased attendance at follow-up consultations. Appreciation of the therapist at the end of treatment was associated with better general functioning, greater motivation (but not better follow-up) and better appreciation of the workshops. These results are difficult to interpret because the trial is not controlled and a multitude of factors, many of which are not measured, are involved. Therefore, no causal link can be established.

We will dwell a little more on the third and last study, one of the rare French studies, that of L. Schiltz. It seems to us that, in contrast to the majority of the other studies, it demonstrates a remarkable method and a desire for rigor. It concerns the identity reconstruction of incarcerated drug addicts.[147] This study is part of a larger group, aiming to explore the effects of art-mediated psychotherapy with people in great precariousness, suffering from stigmatization and social alienation (homeless, long-term unemployed, refugees and asylum seekers, drug addicts in prison or coming out of prison).[138]

96% of the drawings produced by people in a situation of marginalization and exclusion could be classified in one of five categories: type 1: "nostalgia for a lost paradise", type 2: "fascination with the forces of evil", type 3: "graphics and ornamentation", type 4: "escape into the banal", type 5: "fragmentation and dislocation of forms". Types 3 and 4 corresponded to a more pronounced defensive functioning. Type 5 indicated a psychotic process or advanced organic deterioration (none for the prison study). Types 1 and 2 corresponded to a more authentic expression of feelings, whether it was the expression of nostalgia, needs for tenderness and belonging, or depression and destructive tendencies. The analysis of the productions showed that half belonged to group 3 and more than 20% to group 4.

Using a content analysis grid for pictorial production[148] , groupings could be made and resulted in three dimensions: firstly "creativity and formal application linked to a positive atmosphere", secondly "expression of destructive tendencies" and thirdly "abstract content and ornamental graphics". It was noted that for the themes of love, sexuality or religion, group 3 was predominantly represented (indicating defensive functioning).

In practice, the sessions took place in small groups, on a weekly basis, for six months to a year and were accompanied by individual interviews. They were multimodal, combining active music therapy, pictorial and literary expression.

Throughout the evolution, formal indicators were collected in order to document changes. "The pre-test-post-test comparison of the artistic productions made it possible to identify some indications of positive evolution of the capacity of imaginary and symbolic elaboration, appearing as much in the improvement of the stylistic and formal qualities of the productions as in the evolution of the contents in the direction of a more authentic expression of feelings. The convergent evolution of literary and pictorial production (rank correlations between the variables of the content analysis grids for literary and pictorial production) allows us to conclude that the same process of symbolization exists, underlying different modalities of expression."

Several results are detailed with regard to addictions. Relaxation of defensive functioning *(Change in the distribution of types; diversification and appearance of new types in the pictorial production)* ; decrease of the cleavage *(Appearance of depressive themes in the pictorial and literary production, expression of unfulfilled affective needs, appearance of feelings of nostalgia in the pictorial and literary production)*, channelling of archaic aggressiveness *(Change in the ratio of archaic aggressiveness/ elaborated aggressiveness in the texts)*, development of a mature narcissism *(Change in the facets of the Alter Ego in the texts)*, maturation in the objectal domain *(Vision of the other as a differentiated and unfathomable being on the level of the texts)*, socialization *(Improvement of communication and listening skills in group music therapy)*, integration of reality *(Adequate appreciation of one's abilities and limits in the self-evaluation questionnaire)*, work on form *(Integration of musical parameters, creation of complex musical forms, on the level of musical improvisation; artistic elaboration at the level of the texts)*, balance between the ego ideal and the superego *(Appearance of humanitarian and social concerns in the texts)*.

To conclude this part on the therapies by artistic mediation, we can try to draw some broad lines. These therapies are used as adjuvants in different theoretical models, they appear as a tool allowing a better knowledge, a better expression, a better self-esteem. These results are compatible with the idea that one can acquire skills that contribute to fulfilling, to building one's existence in a way that is no longer focused on addictive practices. Theories, methods and techniques vary, and are often combined, without any studies allowing to compare their respective effectiveness.

7. Conclusion

This conclusion will be the occasion to highlight the elements of answer which emerge from our research work. In our opinion, there are consequent links between psychoactive substances, addictions and creativity. We have highlighted a mutual influence which could be exerted at several levels and notably in the field of care. We have also shown that both are part of the same process with common roots, wings and objectives: to modify our emotions, to escape suffering, anxiety, to reinforce our narcissism, to face death, to seek pleasure... Their problems are universal and concern each of us. The pathological addictive process can intervene there: gradually, these functions are *always* filled by the *same* type of practice which becomes, little by little, the only weapon, the only solution.

The problems posed by addictions are complex, they are intimately linked to universal problems which touch the way we fill, the way we build our existence. Beyond being a substitute, artistic practices could allow to acquire skills, capacities, ideas, to consider differently and to better solve these problems. The therapies by artistic mediation could thus contribute to fill the "functions" of the substances.

A brief review of the literature shows that this idea of using art has already been put into practice in the context of art-mediated therapies. The results lack scientific basis, but seem to be in the direction of a better knowledge, a better expression and a better self-esteem.

It would seem appropriate to conduct research that would allow the use of artistic practices for preventive and curative purposes to be considered, to develop new, more methodologically rigorous studies specifying the role and modalities of the use of art-mediated therapies, and to encourage the concrete and valued development of this type of therapy in addictive care structures.

Bibliography

1. Anzieu, D. *Le corps de l'œuvre. Psychoanalytical essays on creative work.* (1981).

2. Runco, M. A. & Jaeger, G. J. The Standard Definition of Creativity. *Creat. Res. J.* **24,** 92-96 (2012).

3. Sternberg, R. J. & Kaufman, J. C. *The Cambridge handbook of creativity* (Cambridge University Press, 2010).

4. Baer, J. & Kaufman, J. C. Bridging generality and specificity: The amusement park theoretical (APT) model of creativity. *Roeper Rev.* **27,** 158-163 (2005).

5. Kaufman, J. C. & Beghetto, R. A. Beyond big and little: The four c model of creativity. *Rev. Gen. Psychol.* **13,** 1-12 (2009).

6. Mednick, S. The associative basis of the creative process. *Psychol. Rev.* **69,** 220 (1962).

7. Wallas, G. *The Art of Thoughts* (1926).

8. Ji, L.-J., Zhang, Z. & Nisbett, R. E. Is It Culture or Is It Language? Examination of Language Effects in Cross-Cultural Research on Categorization. *J. Pers. Soc. Psychol.* **87,** 57-65 (2004).

9. Jung, R. E. The structure of creative cognition in the human brain. *Front. Hum. Neurosci.* **7,** (2013).

10. Fink, A. & Benedek, M. EEG alpha power and creative ideation. *Neurosci. Biobehav. Rev.* **44,** 111-123 (2014).

11. Shamay-Tsoory, S. G., Adler, N., Aharon-Peretz, J., Perry, D. & Mayseless, N. The origins of originality: The neural bases of creative thinking and originality. *Neuropsychologia* **49,** 178-185 (2011).

12. Kischka, U. *et al.* Dopaminergic modulation of semantic network activation. *Neuropsychologia* **34,** 1107-1113 (1996).

13. Pontalis, J.-B. & Laplanche, J. *Vocabulary of psychoanalysis. Under the direction... [of Dr.]... Daniel Lagache* (Presses universitaires de France, 1967).

14. Winnicott, D. W. *Play and reality: the potential space.* (Gallimard, 2002).

15. Aubourg, F. Winnicott and creativity. *Coq-Héron* 21-30 (2003).

16. *Grand dictionnaire de la psychologie.* (1999).

17. Feist, G. J. A Meta-Analysis of Personality in Scientific and Artistic Creativity. *Personal. Soc. Psychol. Rev.* **2,** 290-309 (1998).

18. Batey, M. & Furnham, A. Creativity, Intelligence, and Personality: A Critical Review of the Scattered Literature. *Genet. Soc. Gen. Psychol. Monogr.* **132,** 355-429 (2006).

19. Runco, M. A. *Creativity: Theories and Themes: Research, Development, and Practice.* (Academic Press, 2010).

20. Lang, J.. Genius and madness: reflections on the case of Camille Claudel (1998).

21. Andreasen, N. C. Creativity and mental illness: prevalence rates in writers and their first-degree relatives. *Am. J. Psychiatry* **144,** 12881292 (1987).

22. Kyaga, S. *et al.* Mental illness, suicide and creativity: 40-Year prospective total population study. *J. Psychiatr. Res.* **47,** 83-90 (2013).

23. Baas, M., De Dreu, C. K. W. & Nijstad, B. A. A meta-analysis of 25 years of mood-creativity research: Hedonic tone, activation, or regulatory focus? *Psychol. Bull.* **134,** 779-806 (2008).

24. Silvia, P. J. Creativity and intelligence revisited: A latent variable analysis of Wallach and Kogan (1965). *Creat. Res. J.* **20,** 34-39

(2008).

25. Sligh, A. C., Conners, F. A. & Roskos-Ewoldsen, B. Relation of Creativity to Fluid and Crystallized Intelligence. *J. Creat. Behav.* **39,** 123-136 (2005).

26. Eisenman, R. Creativity, preference for complexity, and physical and mental illness. *Creat. Res. J.* **3,** 231-236 (1990).

27. Zausner, T. When Walls Become Doorways: Creativity, Chaos Theory, and Physical Illness. *Creat. Res. J.* **11,** 21-28 (1998).

28. Hunter, S. T., Bedell, K. E. & Mumford, M. D. Climate for creativity: A quantitative review. *Creat. Res. J.* **19,** 69-90 (2007).

29. Bentham, J. Introduction to the principles of morality and legislation.

30. *Universal Philosophical Encyclopedia.* II: philosophical notions, (1990).

31. *Grand dictionnaire de la philosophie* (Larousse - Gallica, 2003).

32. Loonis, E. Hedonic psychology and addiction: emotions, cognitions, and personality. *E-J. Hedonology* **7,** 84-111 (2007).

33. LeDoux, J. Rethinking the Emotional Brain. *Neuron* **73,** 653-676 (2012).

34. Cabanac, M. Physiological role of pleasure. *Science* **173,** 1103-1107 (1971).

35. Berridge, K. C. & Kringelbach, M. L. Pleasure Systems in the Brain. *Neuron* **86,** 646-664 (2015).

36. Kringelbach, M. L. & Berridge, K. C. Towards a functional neuroanatomy of pleasure and happiness. *Trends Cogn. Sci.* **13,** 479487 (2009).

37. Castro, D. C. & Berridge, K. C. Opioid Hedonic Hotspot in Nucleus Accumbens Shell: Mu, Delta, and Kappa Maps for Enhancement of Sweetness 'Liking' and 'Wanting'. *J. Neurosci.* **34,** 4239-4250 (2014).

38. Kringelbach, M. L., O'Doherty, J., Rolls, E. T. & Andrews, C. Activation of the human orbitofrontal cortex to a liquid food stimulus is correlated with its subjective pleasantness. *Cereb. Cortex* **13,** 10641071 (2003).

39. Rolls, E. T. & Grabenhorst, F. The orbitofrontal cortex and beyond: From affect to decision-making. *Prog. Neurobiol.* **86,** 216-244 (2008).

40. Damasio, A., Damasio, H. & Tranel, D. Persistence of Feelings and Sentience after Bilateral Damage of the Insula. *Cereb. Cortex* **23,** 833846 (2013).

41. Apter, M. J. Reversal theory and personality: A review. *J. Res. Personal.* **18,** 265-288 (1984).

42. Aristotle. in *Ethics to Eudemus* **I,** 45 (Vrin, 1991).

43. Reynolds, S. M. & Berridge, K. C. Emotional environments retune the valence of appetitive versus fearful functions in nucleus accumbens. *Nat. Neurosci.* **11,** 423-425 (2008).

44. Becker, H. S. *Outsiders; studies in the sociology of deviance.* (Free Press of Glencoe, 1963).

45. Chenu, A. & Tassin, J.-P. Pleasure: neurobiological and Freudian conception. *L'Encéphale* **40,** 100-107 (2014).

46. Solomon, R. L. & Corbit, J. D. An opponent-process theory of motivation: I. Temporal dynamics of affect. *Psychol. Rev.* **81,** 119 (1974).

47. Robinson, T. E. & Berridge, K. C. The neural basis of drug craving: An incentive-sensitization theory of addiction. *Brain Res. Rev.* **18,** 247- 291 (1993).

48. Longo, D. L., Volkow, N. D., Koob, G. F. & McLellan, A. T. Neurobiologic Advances from the Brain Disease Model of Addiction. *N. Engl. J. Med.* **374,** 363-371 (2016).

49. Koob, G. F. & Volkow, N. D. Neurocircuitry of addiction. *Neuropsychopharmacology* **35,** 217-238 (2010).

50. Pierce, R. C. & Kumaresan, V. The mesolimbic dopamine system: The final common pathway for the reinforcing effect of drugs of abuse? *Neurosci. Biobehav. Rev.* **30,** 215-238 (2006).

51. Volkow, N. D., Fowler, J. S. & Wang, G.-J. The addicted human brain viewed in the light of imaging studies: brain circuits and treatment strategies. *Neuropharmacology* **47,** 3-13 (2004).

52. Le Moal, M. & Koob, G. F. Drug addiction: Pathways to the disease and pathophysiological perspectives. *Eur. Neuropsychopharmacol.* **17,** 377-393 (2007).

53. Naassila, M. Neurobiology of addiction. In Benyamina A. *Addictions et comorbidités,* Paris, Dunod; pp. 25-54 (2014).

54. Rigaud, A. Psychodynamics. In Benyamina A. *Addictions et comorbidités,* Paris, Dunod; 2014 pp. 67-96 (2014).

55. McDougall, J. The psychic economy of addiction. *Rev. Fr. Psychanal.* **68,** 511-527 (2004).

56. Zuckerman, M. *Behavioral expressions and biosocial bases of sensation seeking* (Cambridge university press, 1994).

57. Karila, L. & Reynaud, M. in *Traité d'addictologie* (Flammarion, 2006).

58. Chakroun, N., Doron, J. & Swendsen, J. Substance use, emotional problems, and personality traits: testing two models of association. *L'Encéphale* **30,** 564-569 (2004).

59. Franques, P., Auriacombe, M. & Tignol, J. Personalities of the drug addict. *L'Encéphale* **26,** 68-78 (2000).

60. Regier DA, Farmer ME, Rae DS & et al. Comorbidity of mental disorders with alcohol and other drug abuse: Results from the epidemiologic catchment area (eca) study. *JAMA* **264,** 2511-2518 (1990).

61. Merikangas, K. R. *et al.* Comorbidity of substance use disorders with mood and anxiety disorders: Results of the international consortium in psychiatric epidemiology. *Addict. Behav.* **23,** 893-907 (1998).

62. Benyamina, A. *Addictions and comorbidities.* (Dunod, 2014).

63. Loonis, E. & Peele, S. A psychosocial approach to addiction still relevant. *Bull. Psychol.* **53,** 215-224 (2000).

64. Pedinielli, J.-L. & Bonnet, A. The contribution of psychoanalysis to the issue of Addiction. *Psychotropes* **14,** 41-54 (2009).

65. Oksanen, A. Addiction and rehabilitation in autobiographical books by rock artists, 1974-2010: Addiction in autobiographical rock books. *Drug Alcohol Rev.* **32,** 53-59 (2013).

66. Milner, M. *L'imaginaire des drogues: de Thomas de Quincey à Henri Michaux* (Gallimard, 2000).

67. Blaise, Mr. 'they wanted to send me to rehab.' From bohemian to surviving artist, the evolution of the figure of the drug addicted musician. *Drug Health Society* **11,** 107-122 (2012).

68. Plucker, J. A., Mcneely, A. & Morgan, C. Controlled Substance-related Beliefs and Use: Relationships to Undergraduates' Creative Personality Features. *J. Creat. Behav.* **43,** 94-101 (2009).

69. Ludwig, A. M. Alcohol input and creative output*. *Br. J. Addict.* **85,** 953-963 (1990).

70. Norlander, T. Inebriation and inspiration? A review of the research on alcohol and creativity. *J. Creat. Behav.* **33,** 22-44 (1999).

71. Kalin, R., McClelland, D. C. & Kahn, M. The effects of male social drinking on fantasy. *J. Pers. Soc. Psychol.* **1,** 441 (1965).

72. Wilsnack, S. C. The effects of social drinking on women's fantasy1. *J. Pers.* **42,** 43-61 (1974).

73. Gustafson, R. & Kallmén, H. akan. The effect of alcohol intoxication on primary and secondary processes in male social drinkers. *Br. J. Addict.* **84,** 1507-1513 (1989).

74. Gustafson, R. & Kallmén, H. Alcohol Effects on Cognitive and Personality Style in Women with Special Reference to Primary and Secondary Process. *Alcohol. Clin. Exp. Res.* **13,** 644-648 (1989).

75. Gustafson, R. & Norlander, T. Effects of Alcohol on Persistent Effort and Deductive Thinking During the Preparation Phase of the Creative Process. *J. Creat. Behav.* **28,** 124-132 (1994).

76. Norlander, T. & Gustafson, R. Effects of Alcohol On Scientific Thought During the Incubation Phase of The Creative Process. *J. Creat. Behav.* **30,** 231-248 (1996).

77. Norlander, T. & Gustafson, R. Effects of Alcohol on a Divergent Figural Fluency Test During the Illumination Phase of the Creative Process. *Creat. Res. J.* **11,** 265-274 (1998).

78. Norlander, T. & Gustafson, R. Effects of Alcohol on Picture Drawing During the Verification Phase of the Creative Process. *Creat. Res. J.* **10,** 355-362 (1997).

79. Block, R. I., Farinpour, R. & Braverman, K. Acute effects of marijuana on cognition: Relationships to chronic effects and smoking techniques. *Pharmacol. Biochem. Behav.* **43,** 907-917 (1992).

80. Curran, V., Brignell, C., Fletcher, S., Middleton, P. & Henry, J. Cognitive and subjective dose-response effects of acute oral Δ 9 -tetrahydrocannabinol (THC) in infrequent cannabis users. *Psychopharmacology (Berl.)* **164,** 61-70 (2002).

81. Sessa, B. Is it time to revisit the role of psychedelic drugs in enhancing human creativity? *J. Psychopharmacol. (Oxf.)* **22,** 821-827 (2008).

82. Janiger, O. & Rios, M. D. de. LSD and Creativity. *J. Psychoactive Drugs* **21,** 129-134 (1989).

83. Carson, S. Creativity and psychopathology: a shared vulnerability model. *Can. J. Psychiatry Rev. Can. Psychiatr.* **56,** 144-153 (2011).

84. Jarosz, A. F., Colflesh, G. J. H. & Wiley, J. Uncorking the muse: Alcohol intoxication facilitates creative problem solving. *Conscious. Cogn.* **21,** 487-493 (2012).

85. Knafo, D. The senses grow skilled in their craving: Thoughts on creativity and addiction. *Psychoanal. Rev.* **95,** 571-595 (2008).

86. Pamart M. *L'Abécédaire de Gilles Deleuze* (TV film, 1995).

87. Day, E. Literary and biographical perspectives on substance use. *Adv. Psychiatr. Treat.* **9,** 62-68 (2003).

88. Carly, M. *Simenon, la vie d'abord* (Editions du CEFAL, 2000).

89. Brenot, P. *Le génie et la folie en peinture, musique, littérature.* (Odile Jacob, 2007).

90. Tolson, G. H. (Jerry) & Cuyjet, M. J. Jazz and substance abuse: Road to creative genius or pathway to premature death. *Int. J. Law Psychiatry* **30,** 530-538 (2007).

91. Sévigné, M. de R.-C. marquise de. *Lettres choisies de Madame de Sévigné a sa fille et a ses amis* (Didier, 1847).

92. Lang, A. R., Verret, L. D. & Watt, C. Drinking and creativity: Objective and subjective effects. *Addict. Behav.* **9,** 395-399 (1984).

93. Lapp, W. M., Collins, R. L. & Izzo, C. V. On the Enhancement of Creativity by Alcohol: Pharmacology or Expectation? *Am. J. Psychol.* **107,** 173 (1994).

94. Hicks, J. A., Pedersen, S. L., Friedman, R. S. & McCarthy, D. M. Expecting innovation: Psychoactive drug primes and the generation of creative solutions. *Exp. Clin. Psychopharmacol.* **19,** 314-320 (2011).

95. Cocteau, J. *Opium: Diary of a detoxification.* (1983).

96. Perpère, A. & Egana, M. *Under the influence: Artists and psychotropic drugs* (2013).

97. Michaux, H. *Knowledge by the chasms.* (1968).

98. Rauch, L. The Poet Syndrome: Opiates, Psychosis and Creativity. *J. Psychoactive Drugs* **32,** 343-349 (2000).

99. Roussillon, R. in *Cliniques de la création* VII (De Boeck Supérieur, 2007).

100. Menger, P.-M. Rationality and uncertainty in the life of the artist. *Année Sociol. 19401948-* **39,** 111-151 (1989).

101. Coulangeon, P. L'expérience de la précarité dans les professions artistiques. Le cas des musiciens interprètes. *Sociol. Art* **5,** 77-110 (2004).

102. Scott, M. E. How stress can affect gifted/creative potential: Ideas to better insure realization of potential. *Creat. Child Adult Q.* (1985).

103. Danielson, C. K. *et al.* Trauma-Related Risk Factors for Substance Abuse Among Male Versus Female Young Adults. *Addict. Behav.* **34,** 395-399 (2009).

104. Lowenstein, W. D. *These dependencies that govern us: How to break free* (Calmann-Lévy, 2005).

105. Baudelaire, C. *Petits Poèmes en prose (Le spleen de Paris).* (1973).

106.Boutet, D. Art as a mode of inquiry and knowledge. (2010).

107 Raskin, R. N. Narcissism and creativity: Are they related? *Psychol. Rep.* **46,** 55-60 (1980).

108 Kohut, H. Forms and transformations of narcissism. *J. Am. Psychoanal. Assoc.* **14,** 243-272 (1966).

109 Weintraub D, Koester J, Potenza MN & et al. Impulse control disorders in parkinson disease: A cross-sectional study of 3090 patients. *Arch. Neurol.* **67,** 589-595 (2010).

110 . Ambermoon, P., Carter, A., Hall, W. D., Dissanayaka, N. N. W. & O'Sullivan, J. D. Impulse control disorders in patients with Parkinson's disease receiving dopamine replacement therapy: evidence and implications for the addictions field: Impulse control disorders in PD patients. *Addiction* **106,** 283-293 (2011).

111 . Bindler, L., Anheim, M., Tranchant, C. & Vidailhet, P. The creativity of the parkinsonian patient. *Ann. Med.-Psychol. Rev. Psychiatr.* **169,** 104-107 (2011).

112 . Inzelberg, R. The awakening of artistic creativity and Parkinson's disease. *Behav. Neurosci.* **127,** 256 (2013).

113 . Canesi, M., Rusconi, M. L., Isaias, I. U. & Pezzoli, G. Artistic productivity and creative thinking in Parkinson's disease: Creativity in Parkinson's disease. *Eur. J. Neurol.* **19,** 468-472 (2012).

114 . Walker, R. H., Warwick, R. & Cercy, S. P. Augmentation of artistic productivity in Parkinson's disease. *Mov. Disord.* **21,** 285-286 (2006).

115 . Granier, F. Art therapy. *Ann. Med.-Psychol. Rev. Psychiatr.* **169,** 680684 (2011).

116 MilenkoviC, S. Scherazade and her 1001 Art therapy stories. *Epistemol. Pract. Res. Art Ther. Luxemb. CRP-Sante Luxemb. Fond Natl. Rech.* (2003).

117 .Klein, J.-P. Art therapy: where it comes from and what it is not. In L'art-thérapie *Que Sais-Je* 9e éd, p.5-43 (2014).

118 . Case, C. & Dalley, T. *The handbook of art therapy.* (Routledge, 2014).

119 . Forrest, G. The problems of dependency and the value of art therapy as a means of treating alcoholism. *Art Psychother.* **2**, 15-43 (1975).

120 Harms, E. Art therapy for the drug addict. *Art Psychother.* **1**, 55-59 (1973).

121 Moore, R. W. Art therapy with substance abusers: A review of the literature. *Arts Psychother.* **10**, 251-260 (1984).

122 Dubois, A.-M. Art therapy and addictions, the example of eating disorders. *Ann. Med.-Psychol. Rev. Psychiatr.* **168**, 538-541 (2010).

123 Johnson, D. R. Introduction to the special issue on creative arts therapies in the treatment of substance abuse. *Arts Psychother.* **17**, 295-298 (1990).

124 Waller. *Art Therapy* (McGraw-Hill Education (UK), 1992).

125 Virshup, E. Group art therapy in a methadone clinic lobby. *J. Subst. Abuse Treat.* **2**, 153-158 (1985).

126 Albert-Puleo, N. Modern psychoanalytic art therapy and its application to drug abuse. *Arts Psychother.* **7**, 43-52 (1980).

127 Horay, B. J. Moving toward gray: Art therapy and ambivalence in substance abuse treatment. *Art Ther.* **23**, 14-22 (2006).

128 Cox, K. L. & Price, K. Breaking through: Incident drawings with adolescent substance abusers. *Arts Psychother.* **17**, 333-337 (1991).

129 Johnson, L. Creative therapies in the treatment of addictions: The art of transforming shame. *Arts Psychother.* **17**, 299-308 (1991).

130 Moffett, L. A. & Bruto, L. Therapeutic theatre with personality- disordered substance abusers: Characters in search of different characters. *Arts Psychother.* **17**, 339-348 (1990).

131 Holt, E. & Kaiser, D. H. The First Step Series: Art therapy for early substance abuse treatment. *Arts Psychother.* **36**, 245-250 (2009).

132 Kaufman, G. H. Art Therapy with the Addicted. *J. Psychoactive Drugs* **13**, 353-

360 (1981).

133 Dickson, C. An evaluation study of art therapy provision in a residential Addiction Treatment Programme (ATP). *Int. J. Art Ther.* **12,** 17-27 (2007).

134 Potocek, J. & Wilder, V. N. Art/movement psychotherapy in the treatment of the chemically dependent patient. *Arts Psychother.* **16,** 99103 (1989).

135 Matto, H., Corcoran, J. & Fassler, A. Integrating solution-focused and art therapies for substance abuse treatment: guidelines for practice. *Arts Psychother.* **30,** 265-272 (2003).

136 Matto, H. A Bio-Behavioral Model of Addiction Treatment: Applying Dual Representation Theory to Craving Management and Relapse Prevention. *Subst. Use Misuse* **40,** 529-541 (2005).

137 Aletraris, L., Paino, M., Edmond, M. B., Roman, P. M. & Bride, B. E. The Use of Art and Music Therapy in Substance Abuse Treatment Programs: *J. Addict. Nurs.* **25,** 190-196 (2014).

138 Schiltz, L., Ciccarello, A. & Ricci-Boyer, L. Being ashamed of oneself. Interest of arts psychotherapies for the rehabilitation of people in social exclusion. In Annales Médico-psychologiques, revue psychiatrique (Vol. 173, No. 8, pp. 681-687). Masson, (2015).

139 Milliken, R. Dance/movement therapy with the substance abuser. *Arts Psychother.* **17,** 309-317 (1990).

140 Reiland, J. D. A preliminary study of dance/movement therapy with field-dependent alcoholic women. *Arts Psychother.* **17,** 349-354 (1990).

141 Fisher, B. Dance/movement therapy: Its use in a 28-day substance abuse program. *Arts Psychother.* **17,** 325-331 (1991).

142 Mays, K. L., Clark, D. L. & Gordon, A. J. Treating Addiction with Tunes: A Systematic Review of Music Therapy for the Treatment of Patients with Addictions. *Subst. Abuse* **29,** 51-59 (2008).

143 Glover, N. M. Play therapy and art therapy for substance abuse clients who have a history of incest victimization. *J. Subst. Abuse Treat.* **16,** 281-287 (1999).

144 Feen-Calllgan, H. The Use of Art Therapy in Treatment Programs to Promote Spiritual Recovery from Addiction. *Art Ther.* **12,** 46-50 (1995).

145 Feen-Calligan, H. The Use of Art Therapy in Detoxification from Chemical Addiction. *Can. Art Ther Assoc. J.* **20,** 16-28 (2007).

146 Ross, S. *et al.* Music Therapy: A Novel Motivational Approach for Dually Diagnosed Patients. *J. Addict. Dis.* **27,** 41-53 (2008).

147 SCHILTZ, L. Can art therapy promote the reconstruction of the identity of incarcerated drug addicts? *Rev. Fr. Francoph. Psychiatr. Psychol. Médicale* **115,** 12-19 (2010).

148 Schiltz, L. Content analysis grids based on the phenomenological-structural approach. *Bull. Société Sci. Médicales Gd. Duché Luxemb.* **2,** 265-280 (2006).

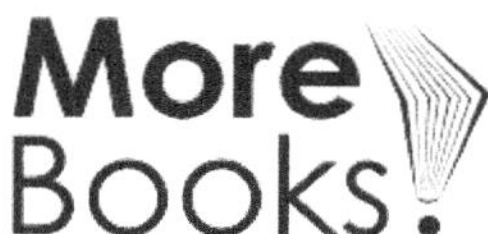

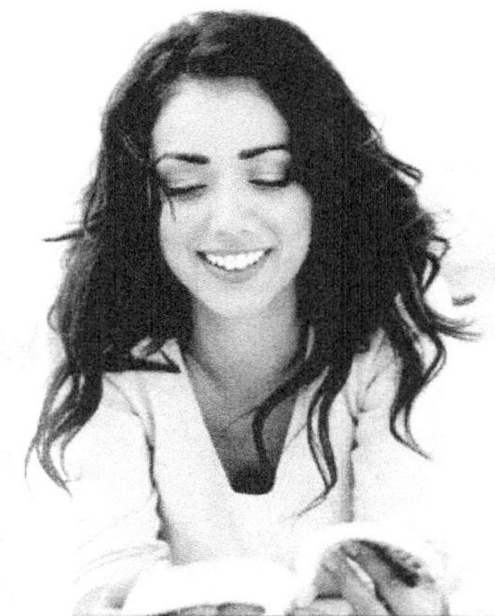

I want morebooks!

Buy your books fast and straightforward online - at one of world's fastest growing online book stores! Environmentally sound due to Print-on-Demand technologies.

Buy your books online at
www.morebooks.shop

Kaufen Sie Ihre Bücher schnell und unkompliziert online – auf einer der am schnellsten wachsenden Buchhandelsplattformen weltweit! Dank Print-On-Demand umwelt- und ressourcenschonend produziert.

Bücher schneller online kaufen
www.morebooks.shop

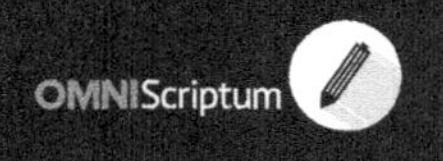

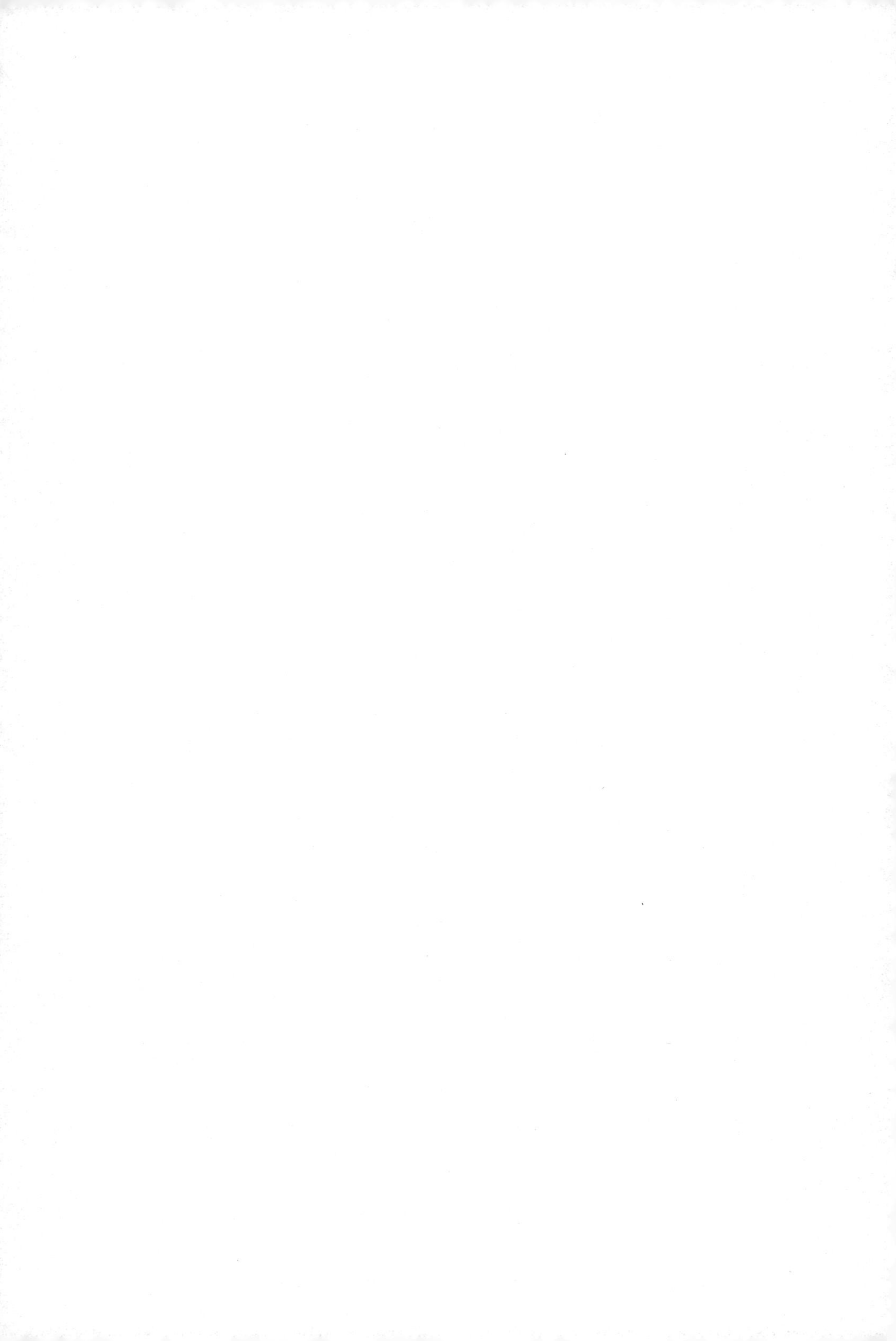

Made in the USA
Monee, IL
07 July 2026

56550842R00066